WHY WE'RE IN PAIN

*Why chronic musculoskeletal pain occurs—
and how it can be prevented, alleviated and eliminated
with Clinical Somatic Education*

SARAH ST. PIERRE, CSE

Copyright 2015 by Sarah St. Pierre

All rights reserved.

ISBN: 0692381619
ISBN-13: 978-0-692-38161-8

Medical disclaimer: This book is not intended as a substitute for the medical advice of physicians. The reader should regularly consult a physician in matters relating to his/her health and particularly with respect to any symptoms that may require diagnosis or medical attention.

As we grow older, our bodies—and our lives—should continue to improve, right up until the very end. I believe that all of us, in our hearts, feel that this is how life really should be lived.

Dr. Thomas Hanna

CONTENTS

	Introduction	1
CHAPTER 1	The Problem of Pain	10

PART ONE
THE SCIENCE OF PAIN

CHAPTER 2	Understanding Pain	25
CHAPTER 3	Why Stress Makes It Worse	53
CHAPTER 4	Natural Pain Relief	69

PART TWO
WHY WE'RE IN PAIN

CHAPTER 5	Developing Habitual Patterns	77
CHAPTER 6	When Our Patterns Cause Pain	104
CHAPTER 7	Why Conventional Treatments Sometimes Work, but Often Don't	120

PART THREE
SOLVING THE MYSTERY

CHAPTER 8	A Century of Exploration	141
CHAPTER 9	Stress and Posture	172
CHAPTER 10	Injury, Handedness and Scoliosis	189
CHAPTER 11	The Daily Grind	197
CHAPTER 12	Personality	201
CHAPTER 13	Automatic Imitation	208
CHAPTER 14	Training Pain	212

PART FOUR
MOVING FORWARD

CHAPTER 15	Clinical Somatic Education	221
CHAPTER 16	Keeping Yourself In (and Out of) Pain	232
CHAPTER 17	Next Steps	253
	Acknowledgments	257
	Illustration Credits	259
	References	261
	Index	295

Introduction

We live in a time of incredible advancement in medical technology. Doctors can give us new hips when ours wear out, new arteries in our hearts to replace clogged ones, and drugs to manage almost any condition. Body parts are being grown in labs, and surgery can be performed by robots controlled by a doctor who is thousands of miles away. It sounds like the stuff of science fiction.

These feats would have been impossible and practically unimaginable just a few centuries ago. Back then, we were more concerned with eliminating viral and bacterial infections that ran rampant through populations, killing thousands of people in a single outbreak. The practice of vaccination, widely considered to be the greatest accomplishment of modern medicine thus far, has turned these epidemics into distant memories for much of the world.

The near elimination of external threats to our health has given us the gift of a longer life span, but it plays a part in a larger trend which is proving to worsen our quality of life. Our successful dominance over our environment has brought with it a sedentary lifestyle, man-made toxins, nutritionally deficient and chemically enhanced food, and new kinds of stress for which we are ill-equipped to handle.

As a result, most of us live relatively long lives during which we encounter a myriad of internal threats. Heart disease, high blood pressure, mental illness, ulcers, cancer, autoimmune disorders, obesity, diabetes, chronic pain and physical degeneration have become the norm. We accept and even assume that we will experience one, if not several of these conditions by the time we reach middle age.

Until very recently in our history, the approach of treating an ailment from the outside in with antibiotics, vaccination or surgery was quite effective and appropriate, given that most threats to our health were coming from outside our body. Regrettably, the medical community has not adjusted its approach to address the vastly different internal threats we face today. To make things worse, we have at our disposal advanced technology that allows pharmaceutical companies to create drugs that keep chronic lifestyle-related conditions under control. These drugs give us the illusion that our conditions are being treated, when in reality they do nothing to address the underlying cause.

The traditional outside-in treatment approach has kept us from recognizing and accepting the fact that we have a tremendous amount of control over our own health. This mental block is exceedingly evident when it comes to chronic pain and physical degeneration. The myth that our bodies will inevitably break down and that we must experience pain as we age is so ingrained in our belief system that few people stop to wonder why this breakdown occurs and if it might be avoidable. As a result, research dollars are spent on developing new drugs that help us manage pain conditions and new surgical techniques that fix worn-out joints, rather than on investigating the underlying cause of musculoskeletal pain and degeneration.

While there are many causes of chronic pain, including cancer, autoimmune conditions and neuropathy, the majority of people who experience pain and physical degeneration do so because of the way that they habitually use their bodies—the way that they stand and move, day in and day out. Their postural and movement habits cause their muscles to be chronically tight and sore, their joints and nerves to be compressed, and their bones to be stressed, often to the point of causing actual damage to the structure of their bodies.

Throughout our lives, we each develop unique ways of standing and moving. While most animals come out of the womb already knowing how to move—picture the lanky foal who awkwardly stands up less than an hour after being born, and is soon trotting around—humans require at least a year of motor learning to reach the same degree of proficiency, and we continue to learn new motor skills and habits throughout our lives. A vast array of factors, including our physical and emotional environment, the way we react to stress, our personality, the injuries we sustain, and sports and other physical training contribute to the motor habits we develop. It is our incredible capacity to learn that sets us apart from all other animals, and that makes it inevitable that we will each acquire a set of motor habits that is entirely unique.

I am describing a learning process with which you are probably familiar: that of developing muscle memory. This term is most often used in the context of sports training, but the ability to form muscle memories is not limited to athletes. Muscle memory pervades our lives, dictating the way that we sit at our desks, allowing us to type and text at lightning-fast speeds, and enabling us to multitask. Most importantly, it allows us to efficiently carry out our daily activities and at the same time be able to focus our conscious mind on more important things. Thousands of years ago, muscle memory allowed us to run after a buffalo while at the same time strategize how to kill the buffalo. Nowadays, it allows us to talk on the phone while we prepare breakfast and do the dishes.

Muscle memory is the result of a learning process that takes place automatically and constantly within our nervous system. This process is critical to our survival and highly beneficial in our daily lives. Without learned motor habits, we would spend all day figuring out how to brush our teeth and get dressed for work. The number of conscious decisions and voluntary movements needed to complete the most basic of tasks would overwhelm us.

Unfortunately, it is easy to develop inefficient and even damaging motor habits. And once learned, these habits feel so natural and automatic that they seem to be innate and unchangeable. They are, in fact, so deeply learned that they are nearly impossible to change unless you understand how your nervous system acquires new motor patterns and maintains levels of muscle tension.

The automatic motor learning process has been part of our neural functioning for as long as we have been a species, yet it is fairly recently in our history that chronic pain and physical degeneration have become such widespread problems. One reason for this is our increasing lifespans. The longer we live, the more time we have to develop motor habits, and the greater the chance that some of the habits we develop will damage our bodies. And the older we get, the more deeply learned our habits become, and the greater impact they have on our health and functioning.

Yet we see children and teenagers who have rounded posture, disc problems, chronic injuries and pain. This brings us to the second reason for our increasing pain: our repetitive and all-too-sedentary lifestyles. Repetitive activities, whether they be playing video games for hours on end or competing in sports, breed habits. Being sedentary is just as detrimental; when our bodies aren't moving, muscles become tight, connective tissue loses elasticity, and pressure is put on joints and nerves. We need not only to keep moving, but also to have variety in our movement.

The third reason we experience so much pain and physical breakdown is the type of stress we deal with in our daily lives. The human nervous system evolved to react to short-term, life-threatening stressors, like being chased by a tiger or being unable to find food. Our current lifestyles are drastically different than they have been for most of our existence. Today, our lives are rarely threatened and we perceive minor events, like traffic or an impending work deadline, to be major crises. Many of these psychological stressors never go away, so our stress response is constantly being activated. As you will learn in this book, stress causes and exacerbates many pain conditions by increasing muscle tension, triggering postural reflexes, and altering the way the brain perceives pain.

If you are like most of my clients, who come to see me after trying everything under the sun to relieve their chronic pain, you know that most of the solutions available for pain relief don't work very well. They aren't effective because they don't address the underlying cause of the problem: the way that we habitually use our bodies. Passive, manual therapies, while often feeling good, simply attempt to fix the pain from the outside in. These therapies incorrectly assume that the structure of the body is the problem. The real issue is how we are functioning, and our functioning can only be changed through an active learning process.

The fact that our function—the way we habitually stand and move—leads to pain and degeneration is not news. Many health professionals recognize this fact, yet they continue to try to fix our musculoskeletal issues by manipulating the structure of our bodies. When their techniques have limited success, our chronic pain and degeneration seem mysterious. They chalk it up to overuse or old age and assume that there is nothing that can be done.

The life-changing news here is the fact that we have the

ability to change the way we stand and move through an active learning process. It is only over the past hundred years or so, with an increased understanding of how our nervous system works combined with a great deal of self-exploration, that people have begun to figure out exactly how to retrain deeply learned muscular patterns and release subconsciously held muscle tension. The techniques of sensory-motor education that have been developed, which you will learn about in Parts Three and Four of this book, will change the way that the medical community and society as a whole think about chronic pain and physical degeneration.

There will come a time—maybe in five years, maybe in fifty—when taking care of our neuromuscular functioning will be akin to eating a healthy diet and exercising. It will be widely accepted that we have just as much of an ability to prevent chronic pain and physical degeneration as we do to prevent heart disease, obesity and diabetes. Getting to this point will require a significant shift in the way we think about our health, as well as fundamental changes in our health care and health insurance systems, but it is only a matter of time.

* * *

I came across a groundbreaking method of sensory-motor education while I was going through a career change and exploring various approaches to movement, yoga and physical therapy. From an intellectual standpoint, I knew immediately that I had happened upon something big. As I began to practice the movement techniques, I felt the injuries and chronic tightness left over from years of intensive ballet training slowly melt away. I gradually became looser, more relaxed, and free from pain and physical discomfort. Looking back on the past seven years, it feels as though my body has been aging backward.

My goal with this book is to explain what causes most musculoskeletal pain and degeneration, and to help people understand that they have the ability to prevent, alleviate and eliminate their pain. I have seen people suffering from back and neck pain, joint pain, sciatica and scoliosis pain for ten or more years become pain-free in a matter of weeks. With such effective techniques available, it is simply not acceptable for people to believe that they have no control over their pain.

In Part One of this book, "The Science of Pain," you'll learn about the reasons and ways the nervous system creates the sensation of pain. In Part Two, "Why We're in Pain," we'll discuss motor learning and how learned motor habits can put us in pain and cause damage to our bodies. Understanding the science of pain sensation and motor learning is an important piece of the puzzle. Knowing the inner workings of your brain and your body is incredibly empowering, and removes the sense of worry and hopelessness about your pain.

In Part Three, "Solving the Mystery," you'll read the stories of pioneering educators who each developed their own method of sensory-motor education. Then we'll delve into the different factors that contribute to our unique motor patterns, from stress and personality to athletic training and injuries. In Part Four, "Moving Forward," we'll talk about ways to keep yourself out of pain, from having lessons with a certified educator to becoming aware of things you may be doing in your daily life that worsen your pain.

This book is for you. No matter who you are, how old you are, or whether or not you have chronic pain. You are human, and this fact makes you susceptible to the cumulative, negative effects of learned motor habits. I hope to educate and inspire you to take control of your musculoskeletal health. It is a process that requires some time and dedication, and it can only be done by you, from the inside. I promise that the payoff—the ability to relieve your own pain, release chronically held muscle tension, and improve your posture and movement—will be well worth the effort you put in.

CHAPTER 1

The Problem of Pain

If you're reading this book, you're likely suffering from chronic pain or know someone who is. Roughly 116 million Americans, or one in three of us, live with chronic pain. It is a debilitating condition which affects our ability to work, exercise, focus, relax, do basic household tasks, get a good night's sleep, and fully enjoy life.

The amount of pain that we have learned to live with is shocking. More than a third of the world's population is in some type of pain, most or all of the time. In the United States, the number of people who live with chronic musculoskeletal pain is almost double the number of people who suffer from heart disease, stroke, cancer, and diabetes combined.

The issue of chronic pain cannot be dismissed or ignored. In addition to the profound effects on quality of life, the amount of money we spend on chronic pain is staggering.

Pain disables five times more people than heart disease, leading to missed work and a substantial drain on our economy. When the medical expenditures of pain care are combined with the decreased productivity and missed work due to pain, the cost to the U.S. is around $600 billion each year. To put this in perspective, heart disease costs the country $444 billion annually, and cancer costs are relatively low at just $125 billion. Yet since chronic pain is not a life-threatening condition, there is little urgency around understanding the underlying cause.

The cost of pain comes out to around $2,000 per person per year—not just for people in pain, but for every single person—living in the United States. A nationwide survey found that most Americans felt pain research should be one of the medical community's highest priorities, and that they would be willing to pay a dollar more per week in taxes in order to increase federal funding of pain research and treatment.

Unfortunately, the funding that is being put into pain research is misdirected toward researching new drugs and treatments that simply mask the sensation of pain. The money spent on pain medications has nearly tripled in recent years, yet the number of people in pain has continued to rise. We are spending more and more money on managing pain, when instead we should be investing in research to uncover the underlying cause of chronic pain. If we do not begin to proactively redirect our money toward understanding the cause of pain and exploring preventative and curative treatments, the number of people suffering from pain, as well as our health care costs, will continue to rise.

Treating Pain

The first stop for many pain sufferers is the drugstore, just as the first step for most doctors is writing a prescription for medication. In 2011, a whopping 238 million prescriptions for narcotic pain medications were filled in the United States. Over the past two decades, prescription rates for these drugs have skyrocketed. The increase is largely due to a few studies published during the 1990s that suggested that opioids, the powerful group of painkillers which includes morphine, codeine, oxycodone and hydrocodone, might not be as addictive as previously thought. This misinformation, combined with a growing demand for treatments for chronic musculoskeletal pain, led doctors to begin more freely prescribing narcotics which had previously been reserved for people who were terminally ill or suffering from severe cancer pain.

Prescription opioids bind to opioid receptors in the brain in the same way that heroin does. The resulting pain relief and sense of euphoria make them not only highly effective but also highly addictive. Just a week or so of regular opioid use leads to a state of drug dependency in which the brain begins to depend on the drug for normal functioning. Repeated exposure to opioids leads to tolerance, a state in which the brain needs increasingly higher dosages to achieve the same pleasurable effects.

The accessibility of prescription opioids, the speed at which they lead to dependency, and the desirable feelings they produce has led to a high rate of abuse. There are now twice as many people dependent on or abusing prescription pain medication as are addicted to cocaine. Three out of four of these people are using medication that was prescribed to someone else, and the vast majority of the drugs are obtained for free from family or friends. The fact that doctors prescribe pain medication so freely likely gives people a false sense of security; they think it's no big deal to give the drugs to a friend or leave them easily accessible in a medicine cabinet. But as availability increased during the 1990s, opioid addiction tripled within just ten years. Opioids quickly became more commonly abused by addicts than tranquilizers and sedatives.

The number of emergency room visits due to abuse of prescription painkillers has more than doubled in the past decade. Larger doses of painkillers, often sought by those who have increased tolerance and addictive behavior, can cause breathing to slow down so much that respiration stops altogether, resulting in a fatal overdose. There are now more overdose deaths involving opioid painkillers than the number of deaths involving cocaine and heroin combined.

The liberal attitude adopted toward opioids in the 1990s, combined with demand from patient advocacy groups for more aggressive treatment of pain, fueled rapid growth in the market for prescription painkillers. Realizing the tremendous opportunity for profit, pharmaceutical companies started developing new and improved formulations of opioids and marketing them heavily. Now that the dangers of abuse, addiction and overdose are being recognized, the drug manufacturers are in a race to develop abuse-resistant drugs. Some of these new drugs are manufactured in such a way as to ensure a slow release of the drug, and others have safeguards such as an outer shell which is difficult to crack. The Food and Drug Administration is beginning to strongly favor drugs that have abuse-resistant properties, and is taking rival products that are more easily abused off the market.

These safety measures are a step in the right direction, but the ease at which prescription painkillers are abused is only part of the problem. The larger issue is that the drugs are being over-prescribed in the first place. Thirty percent of doctors completing their residency have no training on how to prescribe potentially addictive medications, and only one-tenth of one percent of physicians practicing in the U.S. are trained in addiction medicine. In spite of their lack of education, eighty percent of doctors feel they are qualified to identify drug abuse and addictive behavior—and unfortunately, it turns out that they are immensely over-confident. In a 1998 study carried out by the The National Center on Addiction and Substance Abuse at Columbia University, researchers presented a group of physicians with a case history of a 68-year-old woman who had symptoms of prescription drug addiction. Only one percent of the physicians suggested drug abuse as a possible diagnosis.

There is a growing movement toward educating doctors about safe prescription practices and making opioids more difficult to prescribe. Ohio is among a small group of states that have passed laws mandating continuing education for doctors about the safe prescribing of opioids. A few other states such as Washington and New York have strict laws regulating how prescription painkillers get prescribed. In Washington, a doctor prescribing more than 120 mg per day of certain pain medications must get a second opinion from a pain specialist, of which there are few. In New York, refills for some medications are not allowed without a new prescription—which means another visit to the doctor.

While many people favor these trends in legislation because they increase awareness about the risk of addiction, others see potential negative consequences. Older patients and people living in rural areas often have difficulty making the trip to see their doctor in person, which can make getting a refill quite challenging. And there is a fear that more stringent prescription drug laws could produce a whack-a-mole effect, encouraging pain sufferers to turn to illegal drugs. Already, reports show that many people who become addicted to prescription opioids switch over to heroin because of its availability and relatively low cost.

With all of the problems created by over-prescribing, one would hope that at least the people suffering from chronic pain are getting some relief. But it turns out that people find prescription pain medications to be effective in managing their pain just over half the time. Not a great success rate for a treatment that poses so many serious risks.

When drugs don't work, many Americans turn to elective surgery to find some relief from their pain. Increasingly, doctors find that patients are requesting surgery before they have even been examined. And unfortunately, many doctors don't take the time to discuss or encourage non-surgical alternatives such as physical therapy. The sad fact is that doctors make substantially more money doing surgical procedures than by educating their patients on how to take care of themselves. As a result, more and more unnecessary surgeries are performed each year, driving health insurance costs higher.

A prime example of this problem is the surgeries that are performed for back pain. Back pain is the type of pain most frequently experienced by Americans, and it is the leading cause of disability under the age of forty-five. So it's no surprise that back surgery is the most common type of orthopedic surgery, being performed 1.2 million times each year in the U.S. However, it is shocking to note that the number of complex back surgeries performed each year has increased fifteen times in just the past decade. The reason for this drastic increase is threefold. First, doctors earn as much as ten times more for a complex surgery involving spinal fusion than for a simple decompression surgery. Second, both doctors and patients are genuinely attracted to new technology and more aggressive procedures in hopes that they will provide better outcomes. Lastly, patients are demanding fast, effective solutions for their pain, and doctors are limited in what they can offer.

In addition to being the most expensive option for pain relief, surgery has inconsistent and often negative outcomes. In a large cohort study published in 2011, researchers reviewed the records of 1,450 patients in Ohio who had diagnoses of disc degeneration, disc herniation, or radiculopathy and were candidates for spinal fusion. Of the patients who had the surgery, only twenty-six percent had returned to work two years later. Of the patients who didn't have surgery, sixty-seven percent had returned to work. Not only was spinal fusion unsuccessful at relieving pain and reducing disability three-quarters of the time, but the people who elected not to have the surgery fared substantially better than those who did. The study also found a forty-one percent increase in the daily use of opioid pain medications among the patients who had surgery, indicating that surgery may have introduced further pain and led to opioid dependence.

One reason for the high rate of failure in back surgeries is that many people are misdiagnosed as being good candidates for surgery. Often, back pain patients can avoid surgery if they and their doctor take the time to pursue physical rehabilitation. At an annual meeting of the American Academy of Pain Medicine, a panel of doctors led a session entitled "Failed Back Syndrome" in which they discussed the overuse and lack of success of surgery in back pain patients. Dr. Hubert Rosomoff, Chairman Emeritus of the Department of Neurosurgical Surgery and Medical Director of the Comprehensive Pain and Rehabilitation Center at the University of Miami School of Medicine, presented an alarming statistic. When Rosomoff began recommending rehabilitation instead of surgery to his back pain patients, ninety-nine percent of them no longer had indications for surgery just two weeks later.

When the structure of the body is damaged beyond the point that rest and improved movement can allow it to repair itself, surgery is typically the best course of treatment. But when function is the issue—as is the case with most people who have chronic musculoskeletal pain—studies consistently indicate that physical rehabilitation is the better choice. It has a higher rate of success, is less expensive, and has far fewer risks than surgery or medication.

To shift out of the surgery-focused trend we're in, some big changes will have to be made. Doctors need to be reimbursed appropriately for recommending both physical rehabilitation and preventative care. Patients must do their part by educating themselves about their condition and by getting opinions from multiple doctors. Patients also need to recognize that there are no magic pills or surgeries that will cure their pain forever; they need to be willing to put in the work required to take care of themselves on a daily basis.

Living in Pain

Anyone who has been in pain for an extended period of time understands the profound effect it has on their emotional state, ability to focus, and desire to go about regular daily activities. Some pain sufferers are forced to adapt to their condition by making major life changes such as taking disability leave from work, changing jobs, and moving to a home that is easier to manage. Family members and friends who haven't experienced chronic pain can find it hard to sympathize. They should be assured that pain is a very real condition with serious health implications, including an impaired ability to make decisions, increased risk of psychological disorders, and even structural changes to the brain.

Brain imaging studies show that regions of the brain involved in making emotional decisions are also involved in chronic pain. To explore this connection, one study paired chronic back pain patients with healthy control subjects on the Iowa Gambling Task, a card game which measures emotional decision-making abilities. The chronic pain patients performed poorly compared to the control subjects, indicating a correlation between chronic pain and the ability to make emotional decisions.

Another study used functional magnetic resonance imaging to monitor subjects' brain activity while executing a simple visual attention task. Chronic pain patients displayed reduced activity in several areas of the brain that are part of the "default-mode network" or DMN, a group of areas that work together to maintain the active resting state of the brain. Altered DMN activity has been linked to decision-making difficulties as well as depression, anxiety and sleep disturbances—all of which affect chronic pain sufferers.

A whopping eighty-six percent of pain sufferers are unable to get a good night's sleep. This lack of sleep contributes to a state often referred to as the "terrible triad" of suffering, sleeplessness and sadness. Inadequate rest alone is enough to make someone not in pain become irritable. For people with chronic pain, the combination of fatigue, irritability, depression and unrelenting pain becomes a vicious downward cycle which can lead some to desperately resort to overuse of painkillers and unnecessary elective surgeries.

Another major factor affecting the emotional state of pain sufferers is the feeling of having no understanding or control over their pain. Despite all that modern medicine knows about the human body, there is a widespread lack of understanding of pain in the medical community—so much so that eighty-five percent of lower back pain sufferers receive no definitive diagnosis. The lack of a diagnosis often leads patients to develop anxiety and depression around their condition. Studies show a higher rate of depression among patients who have undiagnosed pain than those with diagnosed pain conditions. Research also shows that when people have a sense of control over their pain, their tolerance for pain is increased.

People who suffer from pain for at least six months are more than four times as likely as non-pain sufferers to be diagnosed with depression. And as pain becomes more severe or complex, symptoms of depression worsen. People with two or more areas of pain are six times as likely to be depressed, and people with three or more areas of pain are eight times as likely to be depressed. Compounding the issue is the fact that depression is vastly under-diagnosed, especially in pain patients. At least fifty percent of patients with major depression are not accurately diagnosed by their doctor, and those who present with pain symptoms are even less likely to be diagnosed correctly. Depression alone is the fourth leading cause of disability worldwide, and is projected to be the second leading cause by 2020. Pain and depression share biological pathways and neurotransmitters, and as a result they often coexist, exacerbate one another, and respond to similar treatment. Knowing this, doctors ought to be vigilant about screening for depression when chronic pain is an issue.

Having an understanding of why they are suffering from depression could help many pain patients feel more in control of their condition, and could motivate them to take a more proactive approach in addressing their pain.

New research has shown that chronic pain can affect both the structure and the functioning of the brain, and these changes might help explain some of the cognitive, emotional and behavioral impairments which often accompany pain. Chronic pain patients are shown to have between five and eleven percent less volume than control subjects in the neocortex, the part of the brain responsible for higher functions such as rational thought, language, spatial reasoning, motor control and sensory perception. This decrease in neocortical matter is equivalent to the effect that ten to twenty years of normal aging has on the brain. The effect of chronic pain on brain volume is directly related to the duration of pain, with each year spent in pain resulting in a greater decrease of matter.

The regions of the brain that tend to be most affected are the prefrontal cortex and the right thalamus, both of which are involved in pain perception. The stress that often accompanies chronic pain is a likely contributor to the neurodegeneration, as the stress hormone cortisol has been shown to cause brain cells to wither away and die. Lifestyle changes resulting from chronic pain, such as avoiding physical activity and mentally challenging tasks, may also contribute to the reduction in brain matter.

* * *

Chronic pain has become a large-scale public health issue that dramatically reduces our quality of life and is responsible for a sizable and growing financial drain on the health care system. At the core of the issue is the fact that the medical community does not know how to address the underlying cause of most chronic musculoskeletal pain. Why are drugs and surgery, which are effective roughly fifty percent of the time, our go-to treatments? The answer of "these are the best solutions we have" is simply not good enough anymore.

As you will learn in this book, it is possible to prevent, alleviate and even eliminate most musculoskeletal pain simply by improving the way that we habitually use our bodies. Creating these changes in our habitual motor patterns cannot be achieved with a prescription from a doctor or a surgical procedure; it requires an active learning process that consciously engages the nervous system.

Western medicine is entrenched in its outside-in approach and reliance on pharmaceuticals and technology, and so far the medical community has resisted embracing anything which does not fit into its limited, structural view of health. But as more and more people realize that drugs and surgery aren't solving their problems, we seem to be nearing a tipping point at which a major shift will occur in the way we think about and treat pain. Our musculoskeletal health is in our hands, and the sooner we accept this, the better off we'll be.

PART ONE
THE SCIENCE OF PAIN

CHAPTER 2

Understanding Pain

Gordon McMurray was a psychologist, and he was examining one of his most unusual cases yet. He was administering strong electric shocks to a young woman and she was not reacting. Scalding hot water and a freezing ice bath elicited no reaction either. He went so far as to subject her to acts of torture: inserting a stick up her nostrils, pinching her tendons, and injecting histamine under her skin. Still nothing.

McMurray was amazed to see that the woman's heart rate, blood pressure and respiration remained unchanged during what should have been painful experiences. Certain reflexes were absent as well; she didn't blink when her corneas were touched, and she couldn't recall ever having sneezed or coughed. She could recognize the pressure of a pin prick, but did not withdraw or wince in pain.

The young woman's medical history provided more clues

about her mysterious condition. Once, as a child, she had bitten off the tip of her tongue while chewing food. Another time, she accidentally knelt down on a radiator when looking out a window; she didn't even notice the heat and suffered third-degree burns.

The young woman revealed that after a day at the beach she would have to carefully inspect her feet to make sure there were no cuts. She had been hospitalized many times due to small skin wounds that had gone unnoticed until they became infected. She was embarrassed about her condition and was curious about the reactions to pain that she observed in others.

As she grew older, the woman had begun to experience a great deal of joint damage, and had several orthopedic operations. Her knees, hips and spine were quite inflamed, and the connective tissues and surfaces of her joints suffered damage. It is not surprising to find someone in their eighties in this condition, but this woman was only in her twenties.

Most of us instinctively shift our weight, roll over in bed, and adjust our posture when we feel discomfort in our joints. But this young woman had never felt these protective sensations. So despite multiple surgeries, her joints continued to be worn away because of the way she was standing and moving.

At the age of twenty-nine, the young woman suffered severe infections which could not be brought under control. The dying tissue surrounding her eroded joints was highly susceptible to infection, and lack of blood flow to the joints made it difficult for her immune system to do its job. The bacterial infections which had begun in her joints spread into her bone and bone marrow, resulting in osteomyelitis. During the last month of her life, she reported feeling discomfort, tenderness and even pain in her left hip. Incredibly, an examination of her nervous system after her death showed no abnormalities.

This young woman, known simply as Miss C., is the most well-documented case of a condition known as congenital insensitivity to pain with anhidrosis, or CIPA. There are fewer than sixty documented cases of CIPA in medical literature. CIPA is an autosomal recessive disorder, meaning that a person must get two copies of a specific mutated gene, one from each parent. The gene mutation prevents pain-detecting cells from developing normally, and as a result the person is born without the ability to feel pain or sense temperature.

CIPA patients hurt themselves without realizing it. Self-mutilation is common, not because the patients wish to do damage to themselves for any psychological reason, but simply because they cannot feel the pain that their actions should produce. CIPA patients often bite their fingers, lips, tongue, and insides of their cheeks, as well as do damage to their teeth. There are stories of people who suffer from appendicitis and feel only slight pressure in their stomachs, but are saved by a family member or doctor who understands their condition. And one case study tells the story of a man who walked on his fractured leg until it was completely broken.

Most CIPA patients do not live past the age of three, and

there are extremely few who live past the age of twenty-five. About half of all CIPA deaths are related to the inability to feel pain and the other half are due to overheating. The A in CIPA stands for "anhidrosis," which means that the body is not able to produce sweat. Without this mechanism by which the rest of us naturally cool ourselves off, CIPA patients experience extremely elevated body temperature known as hyperthermia, which can lead to death.

A life without pain might sound very appealing, especially to someone who suffers from chronic pain. But feeling pain is essential to our survival. Most of us learn quickly through experience to avoid harmful or dangerous stimuli because we know that they will elicit the unpleasant sensation of pain. Children with CIPA must be taught things which are obvious to the rest of us, like that they shouldn't bite their fingers, touch hot stoves, and even jump from trees.

As we grow up, pain modifies our behavior without us even realizing it. Yet as adults, we hear messages that contradict our instinct to avoid pain. Coaches tell us to be tough and play through the pain. Doctors tell us that pain is a part of getting older and that we just have to live with it. So our behavior can be modified in the opposite way as well; we can learn to ignore the sensation of pain to the point that we often do structural damage to bodies—much as a CIPA patient would do.

Pain is your nervous system's way of telling you that something is wrong. This usually means that there is actual damage being done to the structure of your body or that damage is likely to occur soon. It can also mean that something is abnormal in the way that your nervous system is processing the sensation of pain. Whatever the cause, your pain needs to be addressed and not ignored.

Nociceptive Pain

Most often, pain occurs when your physical body is being damaged or at risk of being damaged. This type of pain is known as *nociceptive pain*. Pain is classified into three categories, and conveniently they all start with N. The other two types of pain, which we'll cover later in this chapter, are *neuroplastic pain* and *neuropathic pain*. Neuroplastic pain is experienced as a result of adaptive changes in the nervous system, and neuropathic pain is a result of structural damage to the nervous system.

Before we dive into the mechanics of how we feel pain, let's talk about the nervous system as a whole. All human functions, from breathing and digestion to voluntary movement, consciousness and thought, are controlled by the nervous system. The Central Nervous System (CNS) is made up of the brain, brain stem, and spinal cord, and the Peripheral Nervous System (PNS) is made up mainly of peripheral nerves, which extend from the spinal cord to our extremities.

The brain gets to make all the voluntary decisions like where to go for dinner and what shoes to wear. The brain stem controls functions which are essential to life, such as breathing and heart rate. A person can experience brain damage and continue to live as long as their brain stem is intact and functioning correctly. The spinal cord serves as a messenger, carrying signals from the brain and brain stem down to the peripheral nerves, and sending sensory information back up to the brain. The spinal cord also coordinates certain motor reflexes and movement patterns independently of the brain and brain stem. The peripheral nerves are the final piece of the puzzle, delivering messages to and receiving sensory information from the skeletal muscles and organs.

Our nervous system carries out all of its actions through *neurons*, or nerve cells. The approximately one hundred billion neurons in our nervous system receive information, make sense of it, communicate with each other, and send commands. Each neuron is made up of a cell body, dendrites which receive messages from other neurons, and one long axon which sends messages to other neurons.

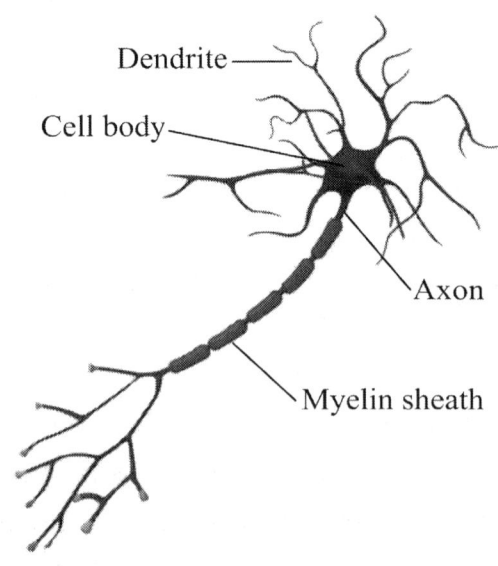

Illustration 1: The Structure of a Neuron

Neurons communicate with each other via electrochemical messages sent through their axons. *Nerves* are bundles of axons which travel from the spinal cord to the extremities (or directly from the brain and brain stem, in the case of cranial nerves). Axons have to be quite long in order to carry messages from the spine all the way to the hands and feet. The longest axon in the body is approximately three feet long. To put this in perspective, if the cell body were the size of a tennis ball, the dendrites would be about thirty-three feet long and the axon would be half a mile long.

Substances called neurotransmitters facilitate the actual transmission of the neurons' messages at the *synapse*, or junction, between the axon of one neuron and the dendrite of another. Over time, as certain neurons communicate with others repeatedly in the same way, neural pathways are formed and strengthened. These pathways create our behavior, habits, and perception of the world around us.

When we feel feel nociceptive pain, two things are taking place. First is nociception, which occurs when damaging stimuli are detected by the peripheral nerves, and the nerves send a message up to the brain saying, "Hey! Our body is being damaged or might possibly be damaged if you don't do something!" Second, when that message reaches the brain, a perceptual process creates the actual sensation of pain. That sensation is a not-so-gentle reminder to your consciousness that something is wrong with your physical body. Interestingly, it's possible for nociception to occur without the sensation of pain, and likewise, we can experience pain even when nociception is not occurring.

Now let's take a more detailed look at how nociception works. The peripheral nerves form a vast, dense network; there are more than a thousand nerve endings in just one square inch of skin. And while we are most often aware of nerve sensation on our skin, nerve endings are present throughout our muscles, joints, blood vessels, and most organs as well. Some of these nerve endings are specialized receptors called nociceptors, a term derived from the Latin word *nocere* which means "to hurt." Most nociceptors respond to all potentially damaging stimuli, but some respond selectively to mechanical stimulation such as strong pressure, thermal changes such as extreme heat or cold, and chemicals such as histamines.

When we encounter a potential physical threat, whether it be an external threat like stepping on a thumbtack or an internal threat like twisting our ankle, our nociceptors react immediately. They sense that their membrane is being bent or stretched and spring into action, sending an electrochemical message up to the brain. If cells actually become damaged, the damaged cells release substances such as proteases, potassium and adenosine triphosphate. These substances chemically activate nociceptors, and the nociceptors in turn send the message to the brain that physical damage has occurred. Nociceptors also release substances called neuropeptides which help to transmit messages being sent to the brain, widen blood vessels to allow for increased blood flow to the injured area, and even stimulate cell growth. So, nociceptors don't just passively receive and transmit information; they also actively change the environment surrounding the injury and facilitate the healing process.

The message that tissue damage is occurring is carried to the brain by two different types of nerve fibers. The first type, called A-delta fibers, carry messages relaying acute pain. These fibers transmit the messages which cause the immediate sensation of pain you feel when you step on a thumbtack or twist your ankle. A-delta fibers are able to carry the pain signal quickly because they are surrounded by a layer of myelin, a substance made up of lipids, protein and water. Myelin acts as insulation around nerve fibers, and the more heavily myelinated a nerve is, the faster it is able to transmit messages.

The second type of nerve fibers which transmit pain signals are called C fibers. Between sixty and seventy percent of all sensory nerves fall into this category. C fibers are unmyelinated, so they transmit signals relatively slowly (at the rate of 1 to 2.5 meters per second, as opposed to the speedy myelinated fibers which transmit messages at rates between 6 and 100 meters per second). C fibers are responsible for transmitting the signals which result in dull, aching, throbbing, long-lasting pain.

Nerves from the skin and the organs enter the spinal cord by the same route, and as a result, information between the two can get mixed up. This cross-talk in the spinal cord can lead to referred pain, a phenomenon that occurs when nociception in one area of the body leads to pain being perceived in another area. For example, someone suffering from a heart attack often feels pain in their neck, shoulders and back instead of in their chest.

Nerve fibers carrying pain signals travel along multiple pathways as they make their ascent to the brain. Some of them follow the spinoreticular tract and synapse with other neurons in the reticular formation of the brain stem. The reticular formation is a network of nerves involved in numerous processes including pain modulation and motor control. From there, sensory information is projected to the rest of the brain to be interpreted. Other nerve fibers follow the spinothalamic tract, traveling up the spinal cord, passing through the brain stem, and finally synapsing in a part of the brain called the thalamus. The thalamus acts as a switchboard, relaying sensory signals to the rest of the brain.

There is not just one area of the brain responsible for perceiving pain. The sensation of pain is created by an interaction of virtually all areas of the brain, including areas which might seem unrelated. And interestingly, new research shows that the parts of the brain involved in creating the experiences of acute versus chronic pain are somewhat different. Chronic pain patients show unique activity in the limbic system and prefrontal cortex, parts of the brain involved in emotions, mood, memory, behavior and decision-making. This activity may represent evidence of the neural changes that cause the transition from acute to chronic pain as well as the emotional and cognitive changes that result from being in chronic pain. Brain imaging studies have even identified patterns of brain activity that are specific to different types of chronic pain.

Nociception and Muscle Pain

The idea that stepping on a thumbtack would cause pain makes sense from an evolutionary point of view; this external threat might actually damage our physical body, so our nervous system wants to warn us immediately when it occurs. But sometimes pain arises from internal sources like chronically tight muscles. Tight muscles can feel achy, sore, and sometimes extremely painful, especially if a muscle is in spasm. Yet it doesn't seem that tight muscles would put our lives in danger. So, why do tight muscles hurt?

Let's start by examining what's happening inside our muscles when they're working. Our brain sends a message to our muscles saying, "We're going running—time to get moving!" In response, our muscles begin contracting and releasing in a coordinated, nearly automatic pattern. In order to contract, our muscles use adenosine triphosphate (ATP) as a source of energy. ATP is a molecule used by the body in numerous physiological functions, from muscular contraction to synthesizing DNA to perceiving taste. It even participates in nociception; recall that ATP gets released by damaged cells and activates nociceptors. Because of its important role in so many processes, ATP is constantly being synthesized and consumed by our bodies in mass volumes.

Muscle fibers store only a few seconds' worth of ATP, so almost immediately, the body must start producing more of its energy source if it wants to keep moving. And as long as our brain continues to send the signal to keep running, our muscles will try their hardest to keep up. When muscles require more energy, the liver changes stored glycogen into glucose and sends it into the bloodstream. The glucose combines with oxygen to create ATP, and water, carbon dioxide and heat are released as waste products. This process, called aerobic metabolism or aerobic respiration, is one of the reasons why we breathe heavily when doing aerobic exercise; our bodies need that extra oxygen in order to produce energy for our muscles.

Sometimes, no matter how hard we breathe, we simply can't take in enough oxygen to keep up with our muscles' energy demands. When there is not enough oxygen being supplied, cells are forced to create energy through a far less efficient process called anaerobic metabolism. In this process, glucose is synthesized into ATP without the help of oxygen, and lactic acid is produced as waste.

As lactic acid is produced, the body quickly breaks it down into lactate and hydrogen ions. The lactate is carried by the blood back to the liver, where it is converted into glucose and either consumed as energy or stored as glycogen for future use. Likewise, the body efficiently takes care of the hydrogen ions with the bicarbonate buffering system. Bicarbonate combines with the hydrogen, forming carbonic acid, which is then converted into water and carbon dioxide. The carbon dioxide is exhaled by the lungs, contributing to our increased rate of breathing.

The only time we feel the negative effects of anaerobic metabolism is when we are exercising so hard that this recycling process can't keep up. It is agreed that the dull ache and burning sensation we feel during strenuous exercise is a result of a buildup of hydrogen ions which activate nociceptors in our muscles. In addition, a variety of waste products increase the acidity in our muscles, making it difficult and sometimes impossible for the muscle fibers to function properly. Acidity and energy depletion lead to muscle fatigue—the state at which we feel like we simply can't go on. If we stop to rest and give our systems a chance to catch up, our muscle pain will slowly fade and our muscle function will be restored.

The way our body produces energy for our muscles provides a natural defense mechanism against over-exertion. Muscle pain and fatigue force us to slow down, preventing us from doing permanent damage to ourselves. So next time you have to take a break due to exhaustion or a burning sensation in your muscles, say a little "thank you" to your body for keeping you in check and preventing you from hurting yourself.

As a side note, there is a difference between the muscle pain felt in an active muscle and the muscle soreness which occurs after a challenging workout. This second type of muscle soreness is referred to as delayed onset muscle soreness (DOMS), and tends to peak around forty-eight hours after exercise. Most research suggests that DOMS is a result of structural cell damage that occurs during strenuous exercise, especially types of exercise which involve eccentric contractions such as downhill running. The damaged cells release substances which help to facilitate the healing process, but unfortunately, some of these substances also activate nociceptors. Consider this soreness another reminder from your body to take it easy because you pushed it a little too hard a couple of days ago. As your muscle cells are repaired, the irritating substances are flushed out of your system, and the soreness goes away.

Now, back to answering our original question of why tight muscles hurt. In normal movement, muscles contract and release, contract and release, over and over again. When muscles release and get a chance to rest, metabolic wastes are flushed out of our muscles, making the pain go away and restoring full function. When we hold our muscles in a constant state of contraction, however, this recycling process never gets to happen.

Muscles that are constantly contracted, or being held in a state of *tonic contraction,* are working very hard even when we're standing still. So as you can imagine, they require a great deal of energy in the form of ATP. But unfortunately, contracted muscles squeeze the blood vessels in the area, restricting blood flow and reducing the amount of oxygen and glucose that can be carried to the working muscle. This compression of the blood vessels is not problem during a *phasic contraction*, in which muscles regularly contract and release. But during a tonic contraction, constant compression of the blood vessels leads to *ischemia,* a condition in which lack of oxygen and nutrients can lead to pain, loss of function, cell damage and even cell death.

Lack of oxygen flow means that cells must use anaerobic metabolism to create energy. In a tonic contraction, this process is constantly happening, even during sleep. Lactic acid is continuously getting produced and being broken down into lactate and hydrogen ions. The constant contraction has the same effect as a strenuous workout; the waste recycling process can't keep up and hydrogen ions build up in the muscle. The hydrogen ions keep activating nociceptors, causing chronic muscle soreness and pain. So if muscle pain resulting from constant contraction is what you are feeling, then your pain should go away when your muscles release and oxygen flow is restored.

Now you understand the mechanical reasons why tight muscles hurt, and as for the evolutionary purpose of this type of pain, consider the consequences of chronically tight muscles. First, lack of blood flow can lead to cell death. Second, tight muscles restrict movement and can limit the ability to defend oneself in a physical attack. Lastly, tight muscles and the dysfunctional movement patterns that go along with them often lead to structural damage to muscles, connective tissues, joints and bones. Considering all the potential damage that tight muscles can cause, it's no wonder that our nervous system wants us to pay attention to them.

Nociception and Inflammation

If it seems like you hear a lot about inflammation, you're right. Inflammation has become the latest buzzword in the health world due to research showing the link between inflammation and many chronic conditions including cancer, heart disease, type 2 diabetes, depression and dementia. Ever since these "diseases of civilization" began to take the place of infectious diseases, researchers have been searching for an equivalent to the germ theory of the nineteenth century which led to ground-breaking advances such as antibiotics, immunization and pasteurization. The medical community may now be converging on a unified theory of chronic disease based on the concept that low-grade systemic inflammation is an underlying and maintaining factor in many chronic lifestyle-related and toxin-induced conditions.

When musculoskeletal pain is the problem, however, the type of inflammation that is typically involved is localized inflammation, which occurs at the site of an injury or infection. When cells of our bodies are being damaged or attacked, whether by bacteria, a thumbtack, or repetitive strain, our immune system is activated. Our immune system does not discriminate between physical trauma and infectious invaders. Proteins called *pattern recognition receptors* can detect both microbial pathogens and physical damage to cells, and the immune system responds in the same way to both types of attack.

When these threats are perceived, the immune system goes into high gear in its effort to remove the harmful stimuli and begin the healing process. Within moments, blood vessels dilate and the increased blood flow makes the area of the injury or infection feel warm and appear red. Capillaries become permeable, allowing white blood cells to move from the blood into the injured area. The movement of immune system cells into the area causes swelling, which helps to isolate the invader or damaged cells from the rest of the body.

Both immune system cells and damaged cells release substances known as inflammatory mediators, which help facilitate the inflammatory process. Some of these mediators activate nociceptors, causing the pain that is felt with inflammation. Immune system cells can spread the inflammatory mediators indiscriminately, so non-affected areas near the injury or infection are sometimes painful as well.

Inflammation that occurs immediately after an injury or infection, called acute inflammation, is a survival mechanism that is necessary for healing to occur. Acute inflammation isolates and disposes of pathogens, allows for damaged cells to be removed from the area, and initiates the healing process. Despite these well-known beneficial effects of inflammation, and the fact that excess use of anti-inflammatory medication is known to slow wound healing, anti-inflammatory drugs continue to be widely over-prescribed. A recent study carried out by researchers at the Cleveland Clinic in Ohio brought some evidence to light which should affect the way that anti-inflammatory drugs are used. The study examined inflammation in muscle injuries, and found that inflammatory cells produce a large amount of insulin-like growth factor, a substance which greatly increases the rate at which muscle cells regenerate. As such, efforts to reduce acute inflammation with anti-inflammatory drugs and ice can be counterproductive to the healing of muscle tissue.

Acute inflammation only continues as long as the damaging stimulus is present. Once the pathogens or damaged cells have been isolated and disposed of, the inflammation response winds down. Remaining cells are repaired, inflammatory mediators degrade, and blood vessels return to normal. All in all, acute inflammation is a good thing. We only run into problems when inflammation becomes chronic.

Chronic inflammation can occur whenever a harmful stimulus remains present for an extended period of time. Chronic, localized inflammation occurs most often as a result of poor body mechanics. If we constantly put unnatural or excessive strain on our knees, for example, we can easily damage our cartilage, tendons and ligaments. In its constant effort to protect us, our immune system will wage war against the damaged cells. The resulting inflammation is one of the causes of joint pain that so many people feel on a regular basis. The inflammation will continue as long as the source of the problem—the habitual movement pattern—is present.

If the movement pattern and resulting inflammation persist, permanent structural damage can occur. Joint tissues are slowly destroyed by both physical wear and tear and the immune system attack. Without these protective tissues, bones rub against each other, causing pain as well as damage to the bone itself. Remaining healthy joint tissue is replaced by tissue which has a different structure. This occurs because fibroblasts, cells that synthesize collagen, are quite active in chronic inflammation. Fibroblasts cause connective tissues in the joint to become thickened and scarred, resulting in loss of function and even deformity of the joint. Imagine—all of this inflammation, pain and structural damage caused by the way we habitually stand and move.

Neuroplastic Pain

If you're past a certain age, a friend or family member has probably encouraged you to do crossword or Sudoku puzzles to keep your mind active. Brain training and "brain fitness" programs are all the rage thanks to research that came out in the 1990s demonstrating that contrary to popular belief, humans are capable of generating new brain cells throughout their lives. The term *neuroplasticity* describes the ability of our brains to change and grow. So if you didn't know it, your brain is plastic, and that's a good thing.

The concept of neuroplasticity has actually been around since the late 1800s, if not earlier. Evidence has been gradually accumulating since then, and over the past twenty years the fact that our brains can adapt—and that we can affect how they adapt—has become widely accepted. Moreover, a great deal of research has shown us that the entire nervous system, from the brain to the spinal cord to the peripheral nerves, can change depending on the input it receives.

Traditionally, it was thought that the nervous system was hard-wired to sense and perceive pain in a predictable, unchanging way. We now know that changes occur within our nervous system that affect the way we experience pain. Pain that we feel as a result of adaptations within our nervous system is referred to as neuroplastic pain.

If inflammatory pain continues for just a day or so, our nervous system begins to adapt to the continued nociceptive input. The inflammatory mediators that are released in response to cell damage not only activate nociceptors, but also increase the sensitivity of nociceptors. So the longer the inflammation continues, or the more times an injury is repeated, the more sensitive the nociceptors become. The resulting state of hyper-sensitivity is called *peripheral sensitization*. This general term describes adaptive changes that occur in the peripheral nervous system which increase the amount of pain we feel.

Peripheral sensitization contributes to conditions known as *hyperalgesia* and *allodynia*. If we experience hyperalgesia, our nociceptors are responding more strongly than usual to potentially damaging stimuli. Our nociceptors are correctly sensing a threat, but they are sensing the threat to be much greater than it actually is, prompting us to let out a blood-curling scream in response to a pinprick instead of a more appropriate "Ouch!" Similar yet distinct is the condition of allodynia, in which we perceive a normally non-painful stimulus to be painful. Brushing a hand against the skin or picking up a warm plate might elicit pain, when under normal circumstances those stimuli would not only not evoke pain, but might feel pleasurable.

Hyperalgesia and allodynia are both enhanced by sensitization of the central nervous system. *Central sensitization* occurs when repeated or sustained activation of nociceptors leads to adaptations in the spinal cord and brain which increase our perception of pain. During inflammation, neurotransmitters and neuropeptides are released which allow for communication of pain signals to the brain. Over time, these substances alter the function and activity of the pathways that the pain signals take to the brain. Neurons in the spinal cord become increasingly responsive to pain signals, and more spinal neurons are recruited to receive input from peripheral nerves. In experiments performed on anesthetized rates, these changes begin to take place just a few hours after a muscle injury.

Similar adaptations take place in the brain. Injury and inflammation make neurons more responsive, and lasting pain leads to an increase in the number of neurons which respond to pain signals. Studies of amputee patients show a positive correlation between the magnitude of pain experienced and the degree of reorganization in the brain. It can be a vicious cycle; the more pain we feel, the more our nervous system adapts, and the more pain we feel as a result of the adaptations.

The sensitization of our central nervous system doesn't just make injured areas feel more painful. When the brain and spinal cord become hypersensitive, they can react strongly to stimuli in areas of the body that are far from the original injury. One study showed that people with chronic neck pain were hypersensitive to electrical stimulation and heat in their legs. In another study, chronic tension headache sufferers were found to be hypersensitive to applied pressure on their fingers. A third study found that people with osteoarthritis were hypersensitive to muscle pain, and experienced increased referred and radiating pain as well.

Both central and peripheral sensitization are believed to play a large role in the transition from acute to chronic pain. Functional adaptations in the brain, spinal cord and peripheral nerves can outlast the original injury and lead to structural changes, which include the sprouting of new nerve endings and the formation of new synapses between neurons. For example, in long-lasting muscle inflammation resulting from damage to muscle fibers, not only do nerves become sensitized, but new nerve endings grow and nerve density increases. And the more nociceptors that exist in an area and can be activated, the more pain we feel. Once structural changes have occurred in the nervous system, pain can persist even if little or no damage is being done to the tissues of the body.

Recognizing the role that sensitization plays in developing chronic pain, researchers are looking for ways to prevent patients from becoming hypersensitive. Their approach involves preventing or reducing pain as soon as possible in order to limit sensitization. One strategy that can be used in surgery is called *pre-emptive analgesia*. It entails administering an analgesic, such as morphine or epidural anesthesia, before an operation in order to reduce postoperative pain. Some studies of pre-emptive analgesia seem quite promising, but most have followed patients for just a short period of time after their surgery. However, one study followed patients for six months after having thoracic surgery and found that the patients who had received an epidural block before surgery had a fifty percent less chance of developing chronic pain than those who had received the epidural block after surgery.

While acute pain serves a crucial evolutionary purpose, chronic pain seems to have no value. It does not protect against tissue damage, nor does it promote healing. Even worse, chronic pain can be self-propagating in that the nervous system adapts to increased nociception by becoming hypersensitive, increasing the amount of pain we feel and leading to further changes in the system. Thankfully, research has shown that in many cases, the changes are reversible and normal functioning can be restored. This shouldn't come as a surprise—our nervous system is plastic, after all.

While we can't change the fact that our nervous system maladaptively responds to pain, we can use this knowledge to reduce our chances of developing chronic pain. When we get injured, have surgery, or develop a chronic ache or pain, we should be cautious about doing things that make the pain worse. This doesn't mean that you should lie on the couch immobile or over-medicate yourself in order to avoid feeling the pain. Movement is necessary for the healing process to happen in an optimal way, and overuse of pain medications can bring about a host of other problems. What is important to understand is that the more often your nociceptors are stimulated, the more sensitization is likely to occur. So, running on an already injured and painful knee will not only damage the joint further, but will also increase your risk of developing chronic pain.

Neuropathic Pain

Sometimes during the course of an injury or illness, nerves can become damaged. Neuropathic pain can be the result of injury to either the peripheral or central nervous system, and is caused by damaged nerves sending incorrect signals to other parts of the nervous system. Symptoms often include tingling, numbness, and shooting or burning pain.

There are more than a hundred potential causes of peripheral nerve damage, including physical trauma, autoimmune disorders, genetic conditions, degenerative diseases, stroke, vitamin deficiencies, infections, toxins, and alcoholism. About thirty percent of peripheral neuropathy cases are linked to diabetes. The reason why neuropathy occurs with diabetes is not completely clear; some theories point to high glucose levels, while others believe decreased blood flow or depletion of metabolites to be the cause.

Peripheral nerves are very good at regenerating after injury, growing on average between one and two millimeters per day. This process, called *neuroregeneration*, can allow nerve sensation to be restored and pain from nerve damage to go away. When injuries are extensive, surgery may be performed to graft portions of healthy sensory nerves onto damaged nerves. Occasionally, an injured nerve can form a *neuroma*, which is an abnormal growth of nerve tissue. While neuromas are generally benign, they can cause significant nerve pain.

Unlike peripheral nerves, damaged nerves in the spinal cord face many challenges. The environment surrounding spinal nerve cells is hostile to regeneration, as it contains proteins which cause nerves to grow in the wrong direction and others which prevent nerve growth. On top of that, spinal nerves must grow in two directions (both toward the brain and toward the periphery), and this added challenge decreases the nerves' chances of success. Scientists at the Mayo Clinic are currently developing a technique that combines stem cells, which produce substances that promote nerve growth, with biodegradable tubing. This method creates a hospitable environment for neural regeneration and allows nerves to grow in the right direction. Another group of researchers at Purdue University in Indiana has successfully restored nerve function to guinea pigs by using a polymer to act as a glue to hold severed spinal nerves together while they heal. While widespread use of these methods is still years away, there is hope for people suffering from pain resulting from spinal nerve damage.

Multiple Mechanisms at Work

While classifying pain into three categories is a useful way to learn about the mechanisms of pain, it is important to understand that in many cases of pain, especially chronic pain, multiple mechanisms are involved. Activation of nociceptors, changes in the nervous system, and actual nerve damage can work together in any combination to produce the unbearable aching, throbbing and burning sensations that keep us awake at night and miserable during the day. As a result, many pain conditions continue to confuse and frustrate the people who suffer from them as well as the medical professionals who do their best to help.

One such example is cancer pain. Chemotherapy drugs are the most likely cause of the neuropathic pain associated with cancer, but radiation, surgery, infections, a tumor pressing on nerves, and chemicals released by a tumor can all contribute to nerve damage as well. A tumor that is large enough to damage nerves will likely damage surrounding tissue, thereby activating nociceptors, and inflammation resulting from the damage will create more pain. And if these causes of pain persist, they will likely to lead to adaptive changes in the nervous system which will enhance and prolong the pain.

The severely painful, debilitating condition known as Complex Regional Pain Syndrome (CRPS) is another example of all three mechanisms of pain working together. With a score of 42 out of 50, CRPS is the most painful condition on the classic McGill pain index, ranking above amputation and natural childbirth. Few studies have been done to determine how many people suffer from CRPS, but best estimates suggest that somewhere between 60,000 and 400,000 Americans have the condition at any given time.

CRPS typically develops after an injury, trauma, surgery or infection. It often begins as pain in an arm or leg and then spreads, sometimes affecting the entire body. The most recent research suggests that CRPS is due to dysfunction of the nervous system on many levels. Nerve damage is a major factor, caused both by the trauma which may have initiated the condition and nerve degeneration which can occur over time. Nerve compression or entrapment that puts direct pressure on a single nerve has been reported to cause CRPS symptoms as well. Maladaptive neuroplasticity also contributes, causing sensitization of nerves and dysregulation of circulation. Along with burning pain, tingling sensations and hypersensitivity, nervous system dysfunction in CRPS patients causes swelling, changes in skin color and temperature, joint stiffness, loss of motor control, tremors, abnormal sweating, and changes in hair and nail growth.

Currently, the most promising drug treatment for CRPS is ketamine, a common general anesthetic. Ketamine works by blocking NMDA receptors, which are a specific type of glutamate receptor. Glutamate is an amino acid which is released in large quantities in response to a prolonged or intense painful stimulus. Over-stimulation of NMDA receptors by glutamate can cause central sensitization, so blocking NMDA receptors can allow the nervous system to return to normal functioning. Interestingly, ketamine can also be used as a treatment for depression. By blocking NMDA receptors, glutamate builds up in the nervous system and stimulates other types of glutamate receptors. This helps the brain to form new synapses and repair the neural damage resulting from stress that is so often present in depression.

Medication, physical therapy and counseling are all recommended for CRPS, and often a combination of these treatments over a period of months or years will yield gradual positive results culminating in near or full recovery. But just as the cause of CRPS is not well understood, patients can recover from the condition mysteriously and miraculously. A population-based study in Olmstead County, Minnesota found that seventy-four percent of CRPS cases resolved over a ten-year period, and often the patients recovered spontaneously.

How the Brain Creates Pain

Pain can be a confusing experience for anyone, and it becomes even more so when we consider how the sensation of pain is created. While pain feels like a bodily experience, that experience is actually created by the brain. The emotional parts of our brain, including the anterior cingulate cortex, the insular cortex and the amygdala, are responsible for the unpleasantness that comes with pain. The more those areas are activated, the worse our experience of pain becomes.

Brain imaging studies have demonstrated this quite clearly by essentially "turning off" the emotional parts of the brain. In one study, researchers hypnotized a group of test subjects and told them that they would feel no pain. When the test subjects and the control subjects dipped their hands into hot water, the sensation-processing part of the brain was activated to the same degree for both groups, showing that nociceptive stimulation was the same. However, the emotional brain areas of the subjects who had been hypnotized did not light up, while those of the control subjects did. The pain stimulation and pain signals sent to the brain were the same for both groups, but the emotional reaction and experience of the pain was quite different as a result of the expectation set by the researchers.

Anticipating pain before it occurs can worsen your experience of pain. Have you ever exclaimed "Ouch!" immediately after stubbing your toe, before actually feeling the pain? You've seen your toe hit the corner of the coffee table, felt the pressure of the corner against your toe, reflexively yanked your foot away, and possibly uttered a four-letter word—all before feeling the sensation of pain. The anticipation of pain, often intensified by the memory of past toe stubs, is enough to make you react as if you are actually feeling pain.

In the next chapter, we'll explore how stress, anxiety, depression and anticipation of pain work together to prolong our pain and make it a heck of a lot worse.

CHAPTER 3

Why Stress Makes It Worse

Humans have been evolving for over three million years. For most of that time, our ancestors lived a nomadic, hunter-gatherer lifestyle, moving with the seasons and following their sources of food. Daily life was focused on physical survival: finding food, preventing and healing from injuries, and defending against attack. We evolved to expertly deal with these acute stressors, automatically engaging all systems of the body to help fight the stressor, and automatically returning to normal functioning when the source of stress was gone.

When we perceive a threat to our survival, our stress response kicks in, temporarily creating a super-powered human capable of lifting a car off an injured person or sprinting faster than we ever have before to outrun an attacker. Our brain's perception of the stressor triggers the release of hormones which prepare us to fight, flee or freeze.

Blood flow, breathing and production of energy for muscles increases. Our blood thickens, beginning the clotting process so that we don't bleed to death if injured. Muscles become tense as they ready for action, and postural reflexes prepare us to either stand up and defend ourselves or curl up into a ball. Functions of the body that are not essential for fighting or fleeing, like digestion, immune response, and sexual arousal slow down to allow the body to devote itself fully to its survival efforts.

Then just as swiftly, as soon as we believe that the source of stress is gone, the functions of the body automatically begin to return to normal. Heart rate and breathing slow down, muscles relax, and the digestive and reproductive systems resume their work. It's almost like nothing ever happened.

Evolution prepared us extremely well for chasing down our dinner and defending against attack. But over the past 10,000 years or so, since our ancestors' development of agriculture provided them with a reliable source of food and allowed them to settle down in one place, our sources of stress have changed. Once our basic needs are met, our sources of stress shift from the physical—those that directly affect our survival—to the psychological. Unfortunately, emotional, social and financial stressors trigger our stress response in the same way that physical stressors do. It all comes down to perception; if we perceive something to be a threat, our stress response is activated. But unlike acute physical stress, from which the systems of our body are quite adept at recovering, psychological stress stays in our mind, constantly activating our stress response.

Short-term physical stress generally has positive effects on the body by stimulating cellular repair and regrowth. It is the long-term activation of the stress response that gets us into trouble. When we constantly worry about work deadlines, debt, relationships, and ironically, our health, our recovery response never kicks in. Blood pressure remains elevated and our blood stays thick, increasing our chances of clots, strokes and heart attacks. We habitually take shallow breaths, inflating our chest instead of our lower belly, and we find ourselves short of breath. Our muscles stay tight all the time, ready for action. These chronically contracted muscles use a great deal of energy, causing us to become fatigued. Stress hormones keep the immune system suppressed, keep blood sugar levels high, and lead to brain cell death. In the end, our response to psychological stress usually causes more damage than any of the sources of stress could have caused in the first place.

When it comes to chronic pain, we are interested specifically in two aspects of the stress response. The first, which is the focus of this chapter, is how chronic stress worsens our experience of pain. The second, which we'll discuss in Part Three, is the way our neuromuscular system responds to stress: by tensing muscles and bringing us into reflexive postures, preparing us to fight or to protect our body.

In the last chapter, we talked about how being in chronic pain leads to adaptive changes in the nervous system that increase pain sensation. We focused on mechanical changes in the structure and the sensitivity of the structures that transmit pain signals to the brain and those that perceive pain in the brain. But mechanics are only part of the story when it comes to our experience of pain. The way we react to pain is actually responsible for the most of the unpleasantness that comes with painful stimuli. And not surprisingly, stress makes us react more strongly to pain signals, worsening our experience of pain.

When we perceive stress, a series of hormones released in the brain triggers our adrenal gland to secrete hormones called *glucocorticoids*, a type of steroid hormone. Glucocorticoids bind to glucocorticoid receptors, which are present in almost every cell in the body, and proceed to do their work. They suppress the immune response so that all of the body's energy can be used to fight the stressor. They also increase and regulate the amount of glucose in the bloodstream, ensuring a constant supply of energy. They even improve our memory of events in which we feel strong emotions. So far, glucocorticoids are sounding pretty good. In fact, synthetic glucocorticoids called *corticosteroids* have been used since the 1950s as medications for a variety of conditions in which the immune system is overactive, such as allergic reactions, asthma, dermatitis, hepatitis, inflammatory bowel disease, joint inflammation, lupus, multiple sclerosis and rheumatoid arthritis.

But as the saying goes, everything in moderation. Prolonged activation of the stress response causes levels of glucocorticoids in the bloodstream to be constantly elevated. Just a few weeks of stress causes neurons, particularly neurons in the hippocampus, a part of the brain involved in memory and learning, to begin to wither away and die. So over time, high glucocorticoid levels can lead to diminished memory and attention. Ironically, the hippocampus plays a role in inhibiting glucocorticoid secretion; so the more stress we experience, the more damage is done to our hippocampus, the less effective it is at regulating glucocorticoid levels, and the more glucocorticoids tend to build up in our system...and so on.

Glucocorticoids have an opposite effect on a part of the brain called the amygdala, and this is where our perception of pain comes into play directly. The amygdala, along with the hippocampus and the rest of the limbic system, helps to process emotional reactions and memory. Prolonged high levels of glucocorticoids actually enhance amygdala function, stimulating neuron growth and making synapses more active and sensitive. Some pain pathways pass through the amygdala, helping to create our emotional reaction to pain. So when the amygdala is overactive, our reactions to pain are intensified, making our pain feel worse than it actually is.

Anxiety

Repeated activation of the stress response can lead to anxiety, a mood disorder characterized by constant worry, nervous behavior and general uneasiness. In rat experiments, artificial stimulation mimicking the effect of glucocorticoids on the amygdala causes rats to develop a condition similar to anxiety. Essentially, anxiety is a heightened level of stress that never goes away.

People with anxiety are always on edge, worrying about things that will most likely never happen. Their heightened anticipation of negative events causes them to overreact to a variety of stimuli, including pain. In laboratory experiments, anxiety patients react more strongly to hot and cold stimuli than control subjects, withdrawing their fingers more quickly and rating their pain higher. Similar results are found when pain-related anxiety is induced healthy subjects, showing that even someone without a generalized anxiety disorder can develop anxiety around a specific type of pain.

Anxiety sufferers also remember their pain as being worse than it actually was. In studies of people undergoing dental procedures, those who have the highest level of anxiety before the procedure not only report higher levels of pain than control subjects, but are also the most likely to overestimate their pain three months later. Sadly, their unrealistic memory of the pain only serves to increase their negative anticipation, making their next dental procedure even more painful.

Studies like these led to research testing the efficacy of anti-anxiety medications such as Valium and Librium for pain relief, and now these drugs are regularly prescribed for people with chronic pain. Anti-anxiety drugs work with the reactive component of pain perception; by slowing down the nervous system and making it less reactive, they reduce our experience of pain.

Stress, memory and pain come together in an anxiety condition called post traumatic stress disorder (PTSD). People most often develop PTSD after an experience that is, or that they perceive to be, threatening to their own or someone else's well-being. The condition may arise from a single experience, such as a car accident, assault or natural disaster, or as a result of repeated exposure to a highly stressful situation, such as combat or long-term abuse. People with PTSD tend to suffer from recurring thoughts and nightmares, forcing them to essentially re-live the traumatic event and experience the stress that came with it over and over. PTSD patients experience higher rates of chronic pain and more intense chronic pain than both control subjects and anxiety patients. Various studies report that up to eighty percent of people with PTSD experience chronic pain, and that the severity of PTSD symptoms correlates directly with the severity of the pain.

Not only do anxiety disorders worsen the experience of pain, but simply being in pain can cause one to develop anxiety. Being in pain is stressful. The pain makes us agitated and reduces our ability to focus and concentrate. We worry about the fact that we can't keep up with normal work and activities, and we worry that the pain won't go away. The pain keeps us up at night, and the lack of adequate rest only serves to increase our stress level. Others often don't understand what we're going through, leading us to feel isolated. Worst of all, we often feel that we have no control over our pain. Research shows that forty-five percent of chronic pain patients develop one or more diagnosable anxiety disorders. And up to fifty percent of people with chronic musculoskeletal pain, serious burn injuries, and other painful pathologies such as fibromyalgia, cancer and AIDS exhibit symptoms of PTSD. In fact, people who experience chronic pain are four times more likely to develop PTSD than those without pain. Chronic pain and anxiety disorders are often mutually maintaining conditions in which each exacerbates the other, creating a downward spiral which makes getting out of pain all the more difficult.

Depression

Imagine a person with anxiety and another with depression. The anxiety sufferer has elevated energy in the form of agitation and nervousness. In contrast, the depression sufferer has lower than average energy, unable to get excited about anything and finding it difficult just to get out of bed. Yet it turns out that stress is instrumental in developing depression, and glucocorticoids are again to blame. Research has shown the correlation between both stressful life events and chronic stress and an increased risk of depression. So despite seeming low energy, depressives with elevated glucocorticoid levels experience a great deal of stress and turmoil; but unlike anxiety sufferers, depressives internalize their stress, causing them to withdraw socially and feel lethargic.

People suffering from depression are often unable to take pleasure in activities they once enjoyed, and stress is part of the reason why. Stress and the resulting release of glucocorticoids affect pleasure pathways in the brain, raising the threshold needed to perceive pleasure. A stressed lab rat temporarily becomes depressed, requiring stronger than normal stimulation of its pleasure pathways to elicit a sense of pleasure. Based on this research, you might guess that people taking synthetic glucocorticoids as medical treatment would experience an increased risk of depression, and you'd be right.

What about serotonin, dopamine and norepinephrine, the famous neurotransmitters that have long been implicated in depression? It turns out that glucocorticoids can affect how much of these substances get produced, how they get broken down, and even the quantity and function of their receptors. Abnormalities in the levels of these three neurotransmitters and how their receptors work play a key role in depression, and for some people, elevated levels of stress hormones are the causative factor. For these people, drugs which lower glucocorticoid secretion and inhibit glucocorticoid receptors have been shown to be effective as anti-depressants.

So now that we have some understanding of the relationship between stress and depression, let's examine how depression affects our experience of pain. While anxiety worsens our experience of pain by increasing anticipation and reactivity, depression worsens pain by intensifying negative emotional reactions. The effects of negative emotions on pain perception can be induced even in healthy control subjects with no pain and no depressive symptoms. One study asked three groups of volunteers to read statements describing positive, neutral or negative moods. The volunteers were then asked to try to experience their assigned mood. When subjected to a painful cold stimulus, the subjects in the negative mood group reported more intense pain than the control group, while the subjects in the positive mood group reported less pain than controls.

Certain parts of the brain are responsible for creating these negative emotions, and these same parts of the brain play a role in creating the unpleasant sensation of pain. One part of the brain that is particularly important in both depression and pain is called the anterior cingulate cortex (ACC), an area of the brain located just in front of the limbic system. When you show people photos of their loved ones who have passed away, brain scans show their ACC lighting up. And simply electronically stimulating the ACC causes people to experience abstract negative emotions. Not surprisingly, depression sufferers tend to have elevated resting levels of activity in their ACC. In cases of debilitating depression, the connections between the ACC and the rest of the brain have been surgically cut, resulting in a decrease of depressive symptoms.

When sensory pain information is sent from the periphery of the body to the brain, the ACC helps to create the unpleasantness of pain by creating a negative emotional state. One brain imaging study showed that the ACC can be essentially turned off by hypnosis, allowing people to be subjected to painful stimuli and feel no pain. Like the study we discussed at the end of the last chapter, a group of test subjects was given a hypnotic suggestion that they would feel no pain. When they dipped their hands in ice water, the sensory parts of the brain that process pain information lit up, but the ACC did not.

The good news is that the pathway connecting sensory pain information and the ACC seems to be highly modifiable. The degree to which the ACC is activated depends largely on our emotional state and our behavior when we react to pain. So can we improve our emotional state, learn to modify our reactions, and reduce our experience of pain? Absolutely.

Recall from earlier in this chapter the role that the amygdala plays in anxiety, and how glucocorticoids elevate amygdala function. Interestingly, activity in the amygdala is elevated in people with depression as well. In anxiety sufferers, the amygdala helps to create the emotional states of fear and anxiety. In depression sufferers, the amygdala creates a sense of sadness. The amygdala in people with depression tends to be overactive all the time, responding to everything with a feeling of sadness and worsening the experience of physical pain.

Just like pain and anxiety, the pain-depression relationship goes both ways; depression worsens pain, chronic pain can cause depression, and the two conditions often maintain and exacerbate each other. Suffering from pain that never goes away is enough to make even the most cheerful person begin to have a negative outlook on life. Combine being in pain with the stress of missing work, the inability to do everyday activities, and feeling socially isolated, and a mood disorder seems almost inevitable. To top it off, people in chronic pain rarely get a full, restful night of sleep. A healthy person feels grumpy when they don't sleep well for a night or two, so just imagine what months or years of inadequate sleep can do to your emotional state.

Numerous studies report that well over half of chronic pain patients suffer episodes of major depression or symptoms of depression. Rates of depression increase predictably with pain symptoms; the longer someone has been in pain, the more intense their pain, and the more areas of pain in their body, the more likely they are to experience depression. Sadly, the symptoms of depression are often overlooked by medical professionals and many pain sufferers go undiagnosed.

A new and interesting link between depression and pain is Substance P, a neurotransmitter that helps to transmit nociceptive information from the PNS to the CNS. When levels of Substance P are lowered or its receptors are blocked, pain is reduced. Research shows that drugs which block Substance P can also be effective anti-depressant medications, and that common anti-depressant drugs can lower levels of Substance P. Why? Because Substance P is often expressed along with and located near the release of serotonin, dopamine and norepinephrine. If you're in pain and Substance P is being secreted to help transmit pain signals, it's likely that serotonin, dopamine and norepinephrine are being secreted too, potentially leading to abnormal levels of these substances. So simply having nociception occurring in your body can increase your risk of depression, even when other emotional and behavioral factors are taken out of the equation. And likewise, suffering from depression is likely to elevate your levels of Substance P, worsening your experience of pain.

Fibromyalgia

Now we come to the most ambiguous pain condition of all: fibromyalgia. While many factors may be involved in developing this condition, the most commonly agreed upon cause is stress.

Fibromyalgia affects at least five million Americans, up to ninety percent of whom are women. Muscle pain and fatigue are the two main symptoms of fibromyalgia. Traditionally, fibromyalgia has been diagnosed based on sensitivity to touch at eleven or more out of eighteen specific tender points on the body. However, in 2010 a new diagnostic approach was adopted which will likely lead to an increase in the number of people diagnosed with the condition. The new criteria are based on how widespread the pain is combined with the severity and duration of the symptoms, which include fatigue, unrefreshing sleep, and cognitive issues. Many disorders such as Lyme disease, hypothyroidism, rheumatoid arthritis, sleep apnea, and lupus have similar symptoms, so when diagnosing fibromyalgia it is important to rule out all other possibilities.

Stressful or traumatic events such as car accidents, abuse, repetitive injures, acute illnesses, and certain chronic diseases have been linked to fibromyalgia. In addition, over half of fibromyalgia patients meet the criteria for PTSD. Many people report having recovered from fibromyalgia by making changes to their lifestyle and reducing their stress level. Stress would certainly explain the fatigue that patients suffer, as well as the muscle pain, which could be the result of both chronic muscular contraction and sensitization of the nervous system.

But fibromyalgia confuses both doctors and patients because other factors besides stress can contribute to developing the condition. Exposure to various toxins can lead to widespread chronic pain, and some fibromyalgia sufferers report full recovery after going through a process of detoxification. And while fibromyalgia can run in families, the genetic links that have been discovered so far are non-specific and simply suggest the possibility that a person might develop the condition at some point.

As you might expect, depression is common among fibromyalgia sufferers. People with fibromyalgia have been found to have decreased activity in opioid receptors in parts of the brain that affect mood and the emotional aspect of pain. Researchers say that this reduced response might explain why fibromyalgia patients are likely to have depression and are less responsive to opioid painkillers.

Stress, the Immune System and Pain

When we think of the immune system, we think of winter colds that leave us curled up on the couch with cough drops, or allergies that make us break out in hives. In fact, pain is probably one of the last things we think of as being related to an increased immune system response. Yet the two often go hand in hand.

Sometimes our immune system gets confused and begins attacking our own healthy cells instead of foreign or damaged cells, resulting in one of the more than eighty recognized autoimmune conditions. Stress tends to make inflammatory autoimmune reactions worse, increasing the pain that goes along with inflammation. And for some people, a period of extreme stress triggers the onset of an autoimmune condition, such as rheumatoid arthritis, lupus, multiple sclerosis, Grave's disease, asthma, celiac disease, psoriasis, ulcerative colitis, or inflammatory bowel disease. The role of stress as an initial trigger is potentially huge; some studies show that up to eighty percent of autoimmune disease sufferers experience severe stress leading up to the onset of their disease.

One of the most common, and arguably the most painful, autoimmune diseases is rheumatoid arthritis (RA), which affects between two and three percent of the world's population. In RA, immune system cells primarily target the joints, causing joints to be swollen, tender, stiff and even warm to the touch. The immune system attacks and slowly breaks down healthy cartilage. Then the connective tissue that lines the joints, called the synovium, grows and invades the cartilage and bone. The result is not only chronic pain, but a great deal of structural damage to the joints.

Once an autoimmune disease has set in, stress often causes relapses or flare-ups of the condition. New research showing that psychological stress triggers an inflammatory response from the immune system indicates at least one reason why: stress leads to inflammation which leads to increased pain. Studies have shown that stressful occurrences predictably lead to increased joint pain within one week in people with rheumatoid arthritis. Sadly, many doctors dismiss stress as a factor in autoimmune diseases because these conditions typically respond well to high doses of corticosteroid medications. So here we have a great example of the effects of acute versus chronic stress. In acute stress, the release of glucocorticoids temporarily suppresses the immune system so that all of our energy can be used to fight the stressor. Suppressing the immune system is a good thing for someone with an autoimmune disease because their immune system is attacking the wrong thing—their body's own cells. High doses of synthetic glucocorticoids simulate our natural response to an acute stressor, suppressing the immune response and giving the autoimmune disease sufferer some relief from their symptoms. In contrast, prolonged periods of stress and repeated stressful experiences cause the immune system to become perpetually overactive, triggering flare-ups and worsening pain.

* * *

At this point you might be feeling a little down. Just reading about stress and pain can be enough to raise your stress level and increase your pain. But don't despair. We'll spend most of Parts Three and Four talking about how to prevent, reduce and eliminate pain. And in the next chapter, I think you'll enjoy learning about our natural pain-reducing mechanisms and how to get a natural high.

CHAPTER 4

Natural Pain Relief

People have been using drugs for thousands of years, seeking out substances that will relieve what ails them or give them an unnatural high. One of the oldest drugs known to man is opium, a highly addictive substance obtained from the dried sap of the opium poppy. Evidence of opium poppies have been found in archaeological sites in Switzerland, France and Spain dating 5500 B.C. and earlier, and Sumerians living in lower Mesopotamia cultivated the plant as early as 3400 B.C. The Sumerians referred to the opium poppy the "joy plant," so they were quite aware of its euphoric effects and likely used it for both medicine and recreation.

Opium made its way west, and by the sixteenth century it was being prescribed as a painkiller. In the early 1800s, chemists isolated two of the active ingredients in opium: the alkaloids known as morphine and codeine. Within twenty years, E. Merck & Company, the German chemical and pharmaceutical company now known simply as Merck, began commercial manufacturing of morphine. Opium and its derivatives were heralded as being a gift from God because they came from nature and were so powerful at relieving pain, reducing anxiety, and inducing a sense of euphoria.

In 1874, English researcher Charles Wright first synthesized heroin by boiling morphine over a stove. People quickly embraced this potent, fast-acting drug. Opioid use was not regulated, and by the end of the century hypodermic syringe sets for personal use were sold in the Sears Roebuck catalog. Abuse of heroin and other opioids became a widespread concern. The Harrison Narcotics Act of 1914 was the first move by the U.S. government to regulate the sale and distribution of opioids, and by 1923 the sale of heroin was banned entirely. The group of drugs once thought to be harmless was now viewed as criminal. Physicians were hesitant to prescribe them, and some patients were undertreated due to the tight controls. Not surprisingly, the black market for opioids flourished. The problem of opioid addiction again reached epidemic levels during the decades following World War II.

During the 1970s, several groups of scientists identified specific nerve endings in the brain that are targeted by opium and its derivatives. These opioid receptors are located throughout the central and peripheral nervous system, but are most concentrated in areas of the brain that process pain information. This groundbreaking find answered the question of how opioids work: by binding to opioid receptors, opioids block the nociceptive information traveling from the spinal cord into the areas of the brain that process pain information.

The discovery of opioid receptors immediately raised another question: why would the brain contain receptors for substances derived from the opium poppy? The obvious answer was that the body must naturally produce substances that are similar in chemical structure to opioids. The race was on to find these substances, and within two years researchers had isolated a class of substances known as endogenous opioids, the most famous of which were named *endorphins* (a contraction of "endogenous," or naturally-occurring, and "morphine"). In addition to blocking pain sensation, endogenous opioids have since been found to play a role in appetite, mood control, immune response, and regulation of sex hormones.

The existence of endogenous opioids also explained a phenomenon known as *stress-induced analgesia*. In contrast to hyperalgesia, the increased sensitivity to pain that we learned about in "Understanding Pain," analgesia is the inability or reduced ability to feel pain. In the 1950s, anesthesiologist Henry Beecher published a study in which he compared pain intensity in wounded World War II soldiers to the civilian population. He found that only thirty-two percent of wounded soldiers, compared to eighty-three percent of civilians with similar injuries, requested narcotics for their pain. In 1977, French neurobiologist Roger Guillemin demonstrated that the pituitary gland releases a certain type of endorphin in response to acute stress. Further research showed the release of other endogenous opioids, particularly *enkephalins*, in response to acute stress. This research explained what Beecher had observed—that when we are experiencing acute stress such as being in combat, we actually feel less pain due to the release of our natural opioids.

Unfortunately for us, the analgesic effects of stress don't last forever. They tend to be short-lived, possibly because our opioids get temporarily depleted. Another important aspect of this phenomenon is that stress-induced analgesia typically occurs when there is an external stressor that takes attention away from the pain—like someone threatening our life, or the need to escape a burning building.

Our natural analgesics serve an evolutionary purpose; they allow us to outrun a tiger even if we're injured. But what about acute stress that is not life-threatening? It turns out that exercise elicits the same stress response, triggering the release of opioids which act in numerous areas of the brain, spinal cord, and peripheral nerves to dull pain and produce a sense of euphoria. While this well-known "runner's high" is a great incentive to exercise, it can numb the pain which should be signaling an injured athlete to stop and rest. Stories abound of athletes like Kerri Strug and Manteo Mitchell who keep going in spite of an injury which, in the absence of opioids, would cause crippling pain.

Looking for a way to get runner's high without actually exerting any effort? Try acupuncture. The ancient Chinese technique of inserting needles into specific points on the body stimulates the release of our natural opioids, providing relief from pain and a variety of other conditions which use opioids as neurotransmitters such as depression, immune system disorders, and sexual dysfunction. While scientists don't yet agree on exactly why inserting needles causes the release of opioids, studies have proven the effect by using a drug called naloxone which blocks opioid receptors. When naloxone is administered, opioids are unable to connect with opioid receptors, and the effects of acupuncture are negated.

There is quite a bit of debate about how acupuncture works. In fact, a number of studies have shown that the precise placement of acupuncture needles is fairly irrelevant. In these studies, "sham acupuncture," in which needles are inserted into random points on the body, proved to be just as effective for relieving pain as traditional acupuncture. Yet other research shows the opposite to be true. Some studies have shown that traditional acupuncture is far more effective than sham acupuncture for both pain and immune system function, and researchers speculate that their results may be explained by the fact that 360 out of 361 acupuncture points in humans are located near major nerves. Stimulating pain pathways and neuro-immune pathways could prove to be the mechanism by which acupuncture works.

Our endogenous opioids help demystify another phenomenon as well: the placebo effect. Placebos, traditionally taking the form of sugar pills, bread pills, or colored water, were often given instead of pharmaceuticals to patients during the nineteenth century as a way to calm and comfort them. The benefits of placebos were quite obvious and widely accepted, but the effects were thought to be psychological in nature, and it was believed that placebos had a stronger effect on patients who were less intelligent and more neurotic.

The placebo effect was linked to the release of opioids in 1978, when a study examined the placebo effect in dental postoperative pain. When patients were given naloxone to block their opioid receptors, the placebos stopped relieving their pain. More recently, brain imaging studies have shown that the release of opioids and the administering of a placebo activate the same areas of the brain. Statistically, the placebo effect accounts for about fifty percent of a medication's effectiveness. So for reasons that are not yet fully understood, simply believing that our pain will go away is enough to stimulate our natural pain-relieving mechanisms.

PART TWO

WHY WE'RE IN PAIN

CHAPTER 5

Developing Habitual Patterns

Learning becomes the greatest and, indeed, the unique feature distinguishing man from the rest of the living universe.

MOSHE FELDENKRAIS

A newborn comes into the world and is immediately overwhelmed by new sensations. The chill of the air, the warmth of his mother's touch, and the roughness of a blanket against his skin. This world is vastly different than his mother's womb. Now there is constant stimulation and seemingly no limit to the space around him.

Not yet able to crawl or walk, the infant explores with his eyes and ears. He recognizes faces and voices, and soon begins to interact by babbling and mimicking facial expressions. Around four months, his brain has developed some ability to gauge where objects are in space. With his newfound depth perception, he begins to reach and grab for anything in his field of vision that seems interesting.

The infant's desire to move toward objects that he can now see, combined with an innate desire to be upright in gravity, motivates him to lift his head off the ground. The muscles in the back of his neck contract, and around five or six months the muscles in his lower back begin to contract as well. Now he can move! Gaining control of the extensor muscles of his neck and back allow the infant to crawl, sit and stand.

At this young age, the little boy is already developing learned movement habits; the motor learning process is constantly at work in his nervous system. It begins with experimentation. Each time he tries to climb the stairs he makes conscious, deliberate choices about how to move his arms and legs, and when something works, he repeats it. Soon he has developed a pattern that works every time: he puts his left hand up on the second step, then his right knee on the first step, then his right hand on the second step, and finally his left foot on the first step. He presses his left foot downward, pushing himself up toward the next step, and then starts the pattern again. With each repetition, the movement pattern becomes more deeply learned. Soon the boy can climb the stairs quickly and easily, with little conscious effort. While the movement pattern that he created and taught himself has become so automatic that it seems to be innate, we know that this is anything but the case.

At birth, the size of the boy's brain was around twelve ounces, only a quarter of what it will weigh when he is fully grown. In contrast, most mammals are born with brains that are already ninety percent of their adult weight. Within weeks or for some, just a few hours after birth, these animals know how to walk and communicate with their species, and they rely largely on "hardwired" reflexes and instincts for their entire lives. As a general rule, the smaller an animal's brain is at birth compared to its adult brain weight, the greater capacity it has to learn and make conscious choices. Chimpanzees' brains are roughly half their adult size at birth, and bottlenose dolphins are a bit smarter, born with forty-two percent of their adult brain weight. Elephants are born with just thirty-five percent of their adult brain weight, giving them an incredible capacity to learn. Like humans, elephants go through a learning period of about ten years before they are considered to be fully mature.

Motor learning is a fundamental part of our problem of chronic pain. Our learned motor patterns, when they are unnatural and maladaptive, are the primary cause of chronic musculoskeletal pain and physical degeneration. But before we dive into the details of how we develop learned motor patterns, let's talk about what compels us to move in the first place.

How We Sense

Movement begins as sensation. We sense that there is dust in our nostrils and reflexively sneeze. We feel hunger and decide to get up and make a sandwich. Even voluntary movement unrelated to what we feel in our bodies, such as the decision to get out of bed and get ready for work, is dependent upon sensation to determine the way that we move; we must be able to sense our body position and detect where objects in our environment are in relation to us. There is a constant feedback loop between the sensory and motor nerves. First we sense what we feel in our body, where we are in space and what is happening in our environment, and then we react accordingly.

In Part One we learned about nociceptors, the nerve endings we sometimes wish we didn't have because they receive information that gets processed into the sensation of pain. There are many other types of nerve endings which receive different sensory information, like that relating to what we see, hear, smell, taste and touch in our external environment, as well as what we sense in our internal environment about our body position, relationship to gravity, and temperature. Some sensory nerves send information to the brain, where it is processed and translated into something meaningful to which we then respond. Other sensory nerves synapse in the spinal cord or brain stem, triggering automatic reflexes like sneezes and postural corrections. Three sensory systems in particular—the visual, vestibular and proprioceptive—play very important roles in determining our movement and posture.

In the eye alone there are over one hundred million photoreceptors, known as rods, cones and ganglion cells, which take in light information. These photoreceptors make up the retina, a layer of tissue which lines the inner surface of the eye. The retina processes light information and sends it via the optic nerve to the brain. Various parts of the brain then use this information to create our perceptions of depth, movement, shape and color, as well as to control our daily sleep and waking cycle.

Our vestibular system, responsible for maintaining our sense of balance, gets information about the movement of the head entirely from its internal environment—the movement of its own hair cells. Within the inner ear is a structure called the vestibular labyrinth, which is made up of the semicircular canals and the otolith organs. When we turn our head, fluid in the semicircular canals moves hair cells located within the canals, and vestibular receptors connected to the hair cells relay information to the brain about how fast and in what direction we're turning. When we move forward or backward, hair cells in the otolith organs are moved, giving vestibular receptors information about our acceleration and deceleration. We process vestibular sensation mainly at a subconscious level, automatically adjusting our head and body position to remain balanced. We are typically unaware of our vestibular system unless it is not functioning normally, such as in the condition of vertigo, or when it is forced to deal with conflicting sources of visual and vestibular information, such as occurs with motion sickness.

Working in tandem with the visual and vestibular systems is the proprioceptive system. Proprioceptors are sensory receptors located in muscles and joints which detect changes in muscle length and in the angle and movement of our joints. Muscle spindles, which sense changes in muscle length, and Golgi tendon organs, which sense the amount of contraction in a muscle, are two examples of proprioceptors. Having an accurate sense of proprioception is critical to maintaining healthy posture, relaxed muscles, and natural, efficient movement patterns. Our brain seamlessly blends information from our visual and vestibular systems with information from our proprioceptive system to give us a sense of balance, body position, and how we are moving through space.

Along with proprioception, the sensations of pain, touch and temperature are known as the somatic senses. Like proprioceptors and nociceptors, nerve endings which sense touch and temperature are spread throughout the body. Mechanoreceptors, which can sense bending and stretching by stimuli as small as .006 mm high and .04 mm wide, detect touch and pressure in the skin, heart, blood vessels, bladder, digestive organs and teeth. Specialized mechanoreceptors work with the brain to perceive variations in types of touch and pressure, allowing us to feel the differences between pressing, pricking, stroking, vibrating, tickling, and scratching. Our thermoreceptors are incredibly sensitive as well, able to detect a change in temperature on the skin of just .01 degree Celcius. When pressure is strong enough or temperature is hot or cold enough to potentially cause damage, our nociceptors are stimulated, and we feel pain.

How We Move

All parts of the nervous system, from the brain to the spinal cord to the peripheral nerves, are involved in motor control. Let's start at the top.

The largest part of the brain is the *cerebrum*, and it is responsible for voluntary action and conscious thought. The *cerebral cortex*, often referred to as simply the cortex, is the outer layer of the cerebrum. Its gray matter is made up mainly of cell bodies, glial cells and capillaries. All areas of the brain located beneath the cortex can be referred to as *subcortical*. One of these subcortical structures is the *cerebellum*, which is responsible for organizing our movement patterns. The *brain stem* extends downward, relaying information between the brain and the spinal cord. The brain stem also controls processes that are most vital to life, including breathing, heart rate, consciousness and body temperature.

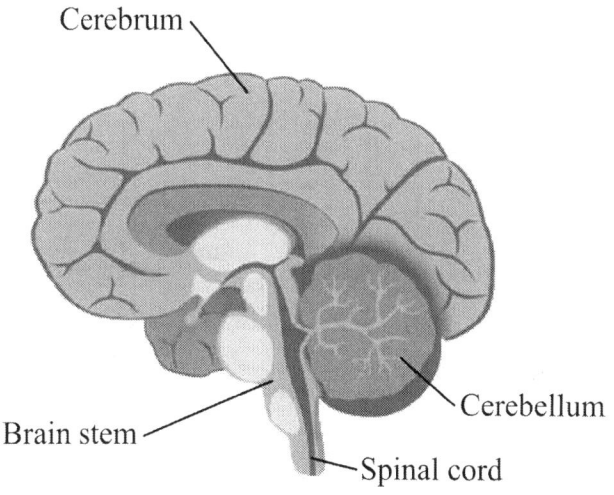

Illustration 2: The Structure of the Brain

Each part of the brain plays a different role in controlling our movement. The cerebrum is responsible for strategy of movement; it is the "big picture" guy. The cerebellum is responsible for tactics; it figures out the sequence of muscle contractions necessary to carry out the movement and how to arrange the movement in time and space. If a person's cerebellum is damaged, they will have difficulty coordinating movement. Finally, the brain stem and spinal cord execute the movement; they automatically adjust our posture to allow for the movement and relay messages which generate the movement.

There are specific areas of the cerebral cortex which process sensory information and control movement, referred to as the *somatosensory cortex* and the *motor cortex*.

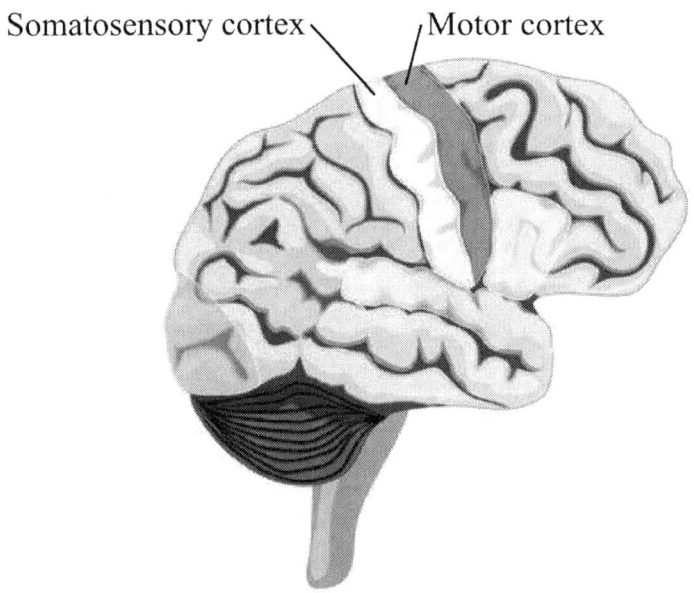

Illustration 3: The Somatosensory and Motor Cortices

Together, these two areas create the shape of a headband, spanning the brain across the head from ear to ear. Each cortex is made up of many smaller areas which are responsible for sensing and controlling different parts of the body, and these areas of the brain can adapt to increased or decreased levels of input and use. For example, a person who had his right hand amputated would use his left hand a great deal, and as a result the areas of his brain that control the movement of and process sensory information from his left hand would increase in size.

For the sake of simplicity, let's classify movements into two types: voluntary and reflexive. Voluntary movements are initiated by the cerebrum; they are movements that we deliberately decide to do and must learn how to execute, such as tying our shoelaces or dancing the rumba. In contrast, reflexive movements occur automatically and subconsciously. Reflexive movements are controlled by the spinal cord or brain stem, depending on what part of the body is involved. Sensory neurons carrying information from our extremities synapse with neurons in the spinal cord or brain stem, and certain sensory information will trigger an automatic response known as a *reflex*. As the reflex occurs, the sensory information continues to travel all the way to the brain, allowing for a voluntary response which may override the reflex.

Reflexes serve a critical evolutionary purpose. Since our nerves are carrying both the sensory and motor signals a much shorter distance—just to the spinal cord or brain stem and back to the extremities, instead of all the way to the brain and back—a great deal of time is saved. Reflexes allow us to respond nearly instantaneously to potentially harmful stimuli. The difference of just a second in reaction time can mean the difference between life and death.

Motor Learning

There are two significant changes that occur in our nervous system as we learn a movement: neural pathways become stronger, and the control and memory of the movement shifts to different areas of the brain.

You may have heard the phrase "neurons that fire together, wire together." This short phrase summarizes the synaptic plasticity theory of learning set forth by Canadian psychologist Donald Hebb in his 1949 book *The Organization of Behavior*. Recall from Part One that neuroplasticity is the ability of the brain to change and grow based on input and use. The concept of neuroplasticity had been previously proposed by others, most notably American psychologists William James and Karl Lashley, and Polish neuroscientist Jerzy Konorski, but it was largely ignored by the scientific community until Hebb brought the concept to the forefront in his groundbreaking book.

In the book, Hebb explains that "synaptic connectivity changes as a function of repetitive firing." In other words, when we repeat an action like swinging a golf club over and over, the neurons involved in controlling that action develop increasingly stronger connections. Not only do existing synapses begin to fire more efficiently, but new synapses are formed as well. As a result, our golf swing becomes more automatic, reliable and forceful the more often we practice. We develop what is known as *muscle memory*.

Despite what the term implies, muscles have no memory of their own—they are controlled by the nervous system. Initially, both voluntary and reflexive movements occur and then cease completely; once we decide to stop moving or the stimulus triggering the reflex is removed, our muscles stop contracting and our body comes to rest. However, when we perform a voluntary movement many times, or if a reflex is stimulated repeatedly, our nervous system notices. And our nervous system likes to be as efficient as possible, because making fast decisions helps us survive. When our nervous system notices that we keep repeating the same movement or posture, it begins to make that movement or posture automatic. As the motor pattern becomes more deeply learned, our brain starts keeping the muscles involved in that pattern partially contracted all the time, and the control of the pattern shifts to different areas of the brain. This process allows the parts of brain responsible for making voluntary decisions to focus on new things which require conscious attention.

In order to demonstrate how lower levels of the brain take over control of practiced movements, researchers from Texas and Iowa did brain scans of people while they learned how to execute a simple finger movement. During the first two weeks of daily practice, the prefrontal cortex—the area of the cerebral cortex that plans complex behavior, makes decisions and focuses attention—was highly interactive with other brain regions. After four weeks of practice, the prefrontal cortex was less active and its connections with other brain regions were weakened. The need for conscious attention was diminished as the subjects mastered their new skill.

Over the four-week test period, activity in the motor cortex and a part of the brain called the *basal ganglia* steadily increased. The basal ganglia is a subcortical cluster of neurons which plays a role in learning, memory, voluntary motor control, and habit formation. The strengthened connections between the basal ganglia and the motor cortex, as well as those between areas within the motor cortex, correlated with an enhancement of movement planning and sequence control and decreasing involvement from the prefrontal cortex.

As movements become learned, not only does control of the movements shift to different areas of the brain, but storage of the motor memories moves as well. For the past four decades, scientists have been debating where specifically in the brain our "muscle memories" are stored. Numerous studies have demonstrated that the cerebellum plays a crucial role in the motor learning process, allowing us to recruit new muscles and control the timing of muscle contractions. Finally in 2006, researchers made an important discovery. By examining eye movements of mice, scientists found that short-term memories created in the cerebellar cortex become long-term memories when they are transferred to the cerebellar nucleus.

The process of motor learning is gradual. The more times we repeat a movement, the more deeply it is learned and the more automatic and less conscious it becomes. The motor learning process is also subject to many factors such as how frequently a movement is practiced and whether or not conflicting movement patterns have been learned before or are being learned concurrently.

Thanks to research on the efficacy of visualization

techniques, we know that we can practice our motor skills and strengthen our muscle memory without actually moving. When we simply imagine ourselves performing a certain task, our brain functions in much the same way as if we are physically carrying out the action. Brain scans show that we go through the same planning and preparation phases, then stop before activating the primary motor cortex.

As a side note, visualization techniques offer great opportunities for athletes and performers, allowing them to practice with no sensory distractions, physical limitations or risk of injury. In fact, an experiment carried out by Russian coaches leading up to the 1980 Olympics showed that not only does visualization work, but it can be more effective than physical training. The coaches separated their athletes into four groups: the first did 100% physical training, the second did 75% physical training and 25% visualization, the third did 50% physical training and 50% visualization, and the fourth did 25% physical training and 75% visualization. Remarkably, the group of athletes that showed the greatest improvement in performance was the fourth group.

Learned movement patterns can remain with us for long periods of time even if they are not actively practiced. While synaptic connections will weaken, some vestiges of the neural pathways remain, and the memory of how to execute a movement can be stored. One study found that people retained typing skills after two consecutive twenty-five year periods of not typing at all. Other research has shown that the ability to juggle, drive and solve mazes can be quickly remembered and reinstated after many years of not being practiced. As the saying goes, it's just like riding a bike.

Despite the potential permanence of our learned motor skills, we do have the ability to learn new movement patterns well enough that they can override old ones. A wonderful example of this learning ability is golfer Tiger Woods, who has deconstructed and reconstructed his swing not once, not twice, but three times in less than two decades. Ever the perfectionist, Woods seems to take great pleasure in harnessing his analytical and kinesthetic skills in pursuit of the perfect swing.

We can learn a important lesson by observing what Woods went through the first time he changed his swing. Shortly after winning the 1997 Masters Tournament by a record twelve strokes, Woods approached his then-coach Butch Harmon about the possibility of improving his swing. Harmon agreed that it was possible, but cautioned Woods that it would be difficult to play competitively while making the changes. Woods refused to listen, insisting that he was capable of implementing the new swing while continuing to compete. He went on to have one of his worst seasons ever, entering a famous slump during the second half of 1997 and winning only one tournament in 1998.

Harmon knew what he was talking about. Weakening the grip, adjusting the takeaway, raising the left arm on the backswing, changing the clubhead angle, and coordinating the timing of the arms and hips were too many changes to make all at once. Harmon also understood that trying to learn how to swing a club in this new way would be virtually impossible while under the pressure of competition; this was why so many other golfers had failed in their attempts to change their swing.

When under stress, our nervous system will automatically choose to act in whatever way is fastest. The movement pattern that is most deeply learned requires the least amount of conscious thought, and therefore the nervous system will be able to carry it out most efficiently. This is why Woods ran into trouble during the 1998 season. He was trying to use his new swing, but it was still tentative and unreliable; not yet well-learned enough to be ready for the pressure of competition. Undoubtedly, the stress was causing him to automatically revert to his old swing, possibly creating some sort of hybrid of the two swings, as well as a great deal of frustration.

Harmon finally convinced Woods to take a year off from playing competitively so that he could learn his new swing from the ground up, one element at a time. Away from the pressure of competition, Woods was able to practice the new swing slowly and consciously—the only way that muscle memory can truly be changed. With repeated practice of a new movement pattern in a non-stressful environment where the old pattern will not be triggered, a new pattern can eventually become stronger and more efficient than the old one. Finally, we can get to the point where the new pattern automatically kicks in when we are under pressure.

It was at this point, just before the Byron Nelson Championship in May of 1999, that Woods famously called Harmon and said, "I got it." Over the next two seasons, Woods won seventeen PGA Tour events, including the 2000

U.S. Open Championship which he won by a record-setting fifteen strokes. This win was the first in a streak of four straight consecutive wins in the four major golf tournaments. From August 1999 to September 2004, Woods was ranked the number one golfer in the world. The time and effort it took to change his swing had been well worth it, and Woods repeated the process again in 2004 and 2010.

Losing Control, Sensation and Awareness

The process of acquiring muscle memory is not limited to athletes, nor is it limited to the learning of complex movement patterns like swinging a golf club. The same learning process is going on within your nervous system, all the time, every day of your entire life, even if you sit at a desk all day and go home and watch TV at night. Some people consciously choose to work with their muscle memory, actively training and retraining their motor patterns in pursuit of a goal. But most of us are unaware that that we are engaged in a constant process of subconsciously reinforcing old movement patterns and learning new ones.

The automatic motor learning process is innate in all of us, and it serves an important evolutionary purpose. Take the example of an infant learning how to walk. He must first focus all his conscious attention on figuring out how to shift his weight to his left side in order to lift his right foot up and take a step. Each time he takes a step, the neural pathways controlling his movements become stronger. Gradually, the control of his walking movements shifts away from his prefrontal cortex, and the infant is able to focus his conscious attention on other tasks while walking around effortlessly. You can imagine how critical muscle memory was to our survival hundreds of thousands of years ago. Back then, only the fit survived, and the ability to move quickly and automatically under stress often meant the difference between life and death.

For most of us today, our survival is not so dependent on being able to move quickly. However, the process of learning and automating movement patterns is hardwired into our nervous system, so it occurs whether we want it to or not. And for the most part, acquiring muscle memory is an incredible ability which we would not want to live without. The key to avoiding problems is that we need to become aware of when we are learning habits which might damage our body or lead to chronic pain.

Our brain wants to help us be as efficient as possible, so it will remember any movement or posture which we choose to repeat—even if the movement or posture is unnatural and could potentially cause pain and damage over time. To illustrate this point I'll use an example to which many of us can relate: that of sitting and working at a computer.

Let's pretend that you have just started a new job, and it is your first ever desk job. All of a sudden you'll be spending most of your waking hours sitting at a desk, working at a computer. Let's also pretend that you are a bit nearsighted. Each time you sit down to work at the computer, you reach your head and neck forward a little bit in order to see the screen better. Then you lift up your hands, bringing your arms forward and rotating them inward so that you can type on the keyboard.

I'd like you to really feel what it is like to be in this position. Wherever you are, please read the next few paragraphs and then put your book down so that you can try this exercise.

Sit up straight and tall with your feet on the ground right below or in front of your knees, head sitting easily on the top of your spine, eyes looking forward, and arms hanging loosely by your sides. Now, bring your head forward a bit as though you wanted to see a computer screen better, and as you do this, pay attention to what muscles you feel contracting. Did you feel where the contraction is happening? If not, do the movement again. You might have kept your torso stiff and just craned your neck forward using your neck muscles. Or you might have contracted your abdominal muscles, tucking your pelvis under and rounding your back. Most likely, you did some combination of these two actions. Repeat the movement again, feeling your pattern of muscular contraction as you bring your head forward, and feeling the release as you go back to your neutral starting posture.

Now bring your arms up in front of you and rotate your hands inward as if you are going to type on a keyboard, and as you do so, notice what muscles are working. If it's hard to feel this one, relax and start over, and try moving very slowly. You should feel your pectoral muscles as well as your biceps muscles contracting as you come into the typing position.

Each time you sit down to work at your new job, your neck muscles, abdominals, pectorals and biceps all contract to bring you into your typing position. At first, this position is new to you and it will likely feel uncomfortable and tiring; you will instinctively relax back in your chair every few minutes, and subconsciously find reasons to get up and walk around.

But day after day, you come to work and repeat this posture. "Hey," says your nervous system, "she seems to like sitting this way. Let's help her out and just keep her in this posture all the time!" Really, your nervous system is trying to be helpful. So it sends the message to your neck muscles, abdominals, pectorals and biceps to stay a little bit contracted in this specific pattern all the time. The control of this posture begins to shift away from your prefrontal cortex into lower brain regions where it can be controlled automatically and subconsciously. You become accustomed to the feeling of being in this posture, and it feels more and more comfortable every day. Now you can stop wasting conscious attention on your posture and focus on your work.

When the brain sends the message to a muscle to contract, the message is sent via an upper motor neuron, which synapses on a lower motor neuron in the spinal cord. The lower motor neuron then carries the signal to the muscle fibers to tell them to contract. The brain can only send one type of signal to a muscle, and that is to contract; it cannot send an active message to release. When an action is complete and the message to contract is not being sent anymore, muscles should automatically relax back to their full resting length.

Unfortunately, as you just learned, it is very easy to form muscular habits which involve keeping certain muscles a little bit contracted all the time. As you learned in Part One, this chronic contraction leads to the constant buildup of hydrogen ions which activate your nociceptors, causing pain. Now you can begin to see how our natural learning process of developing muscle memory can so easily lead to discomfort, poor posture and pain.

Loss of voluntary, conscious control of our muscles is only one piece of the puzzle. Loss of sensation and sensory awareness also play a large role in developing habitual motor patterns. As a stimulus is repeated, most of our sensory systems become less responsive. This process is known as *sensory adaptation.*

We've already learned that we become more sensitive to pain the more our nociceptors are activated, but our pain processing system is one of the exceptions. In general, activity in sensory systems is highest during and immediately after a new stimulus is presented. Within a short period of time our sensory receptors return to their normal resting state, even if the stimulus is still present.

Imagine going swimming in cool ocean water. When you first dip your toes into the water, it feels quite chilly. If you stand there for a minute, letting the waves lap over your feet, you get used to the temperature and it begins to feel comfortable. Wading in deeper, you experience this phenomenon each time the water comes into contact with a new part of your body. Soon you are fully submerged, your thermoreceptors have returned to their resting state, and the water actually feels warm.

We quickly adapt in a similar way to new sensations of

touch, sound, smell and taste. Wearing a new bracelet can be bothersome and distracting until you get used to the sensation of the metal touching your wrist. A repetitive sound like a car alarm is at first annoying, but quickly fades into the background. An unpleasant odor can be overwhelming as you enter a room, but within minutes you barely notice it. A sugary drink seems too sweet until you have taken several sips and become used to the taste.

When it comes to learned movement patterns, we're concerned with the adaptation of our vestibular system and our proprioceptive system. Our vestibular system adapts when we are in motion at the same speed for longer than a few moments; so when we are flying in an airplane at 600 miles per hour, we feel like we're sitting still. Likewise, if we tip our head slightly forward or to the side, after a while the tilted position begins to feel normal. This adaptation is a function of both the vestibular and proprioceptive systems.

As I mentioned earlier in this chapter, proprioceptors are sensory receptors located in our muscles and joints. The proprioceptors in our joints detect changes in the angle, direction and speed of movement in our joints. These proprioceptors adapt quickly; they are very good at sensing changes in our joint position as we move, but they give us very little information about the resting position of our joints. This adaptability is helpful when we are in motion, but allows us to get comfortable in unnatural resting positions—like slouched forward at a computer.

Proprioceptors located within our muscles also allow us to get comfortable in unnatural positions. These proprioceptors, which sense changes in muscle length, are formally called muscle spindles but often referred to as stretch receptors because they can sense when a muscle is being stretched.

Muscle spindles play a critical role in allowing us to maintain upright posture and control of our muscles. In fact, mice without these proprioceptors have abnormal posture and are not able to support their own weight. Humans have evolved to have a particularly high density of muscle spindles in the muscles of our neck, giving us a great deal of control over the support of our head. And as it turns out, muscle spindles are involved in the process of developing damaging motor patterns and chronic pain.

Recall from a few pages ago that a lower motor neuron carries the message from the spinal cord to the muscle telling the muscle fibers to contract. There are two types of lower motor neurons: alpha motor neurons and gamma motor neurons. Alpha motor neurons innervate extrafusal muscle fibers, the type of fibers which make up the bulk of all skeletal muscles, while gamma motor neurons innervate intrafusal muscle fibers.

Muscle spindles, located in the belly of most skeletal muscles, are made up of specialized intrafusal muscle fibers wrapped in a fibrous capsule. When the extrafusal fibers of a muscle are lengthened, the intrafusal fibers of the muscle spindle can't help but lengthen as well. Axons of sensory neurons are wrapped around the muscle spindle in order to sense its length and the muscle's length. These sensory axons, known as Ia axons, are among those with the thickest myelin sheath of all axons in the body, allowing the messages being sent through them to travel at speeds up to around one hundred meters per second.

When a muscle is stretched, the sensory axons wrapped around the muscle spindle sense the increase in length, and send this information to the alpha motor neuron. The alpha motor neuron then immediately sends the message to the extrafusal muscle fibers to contract in order to protect the muscle from being torn. This nearly instantaneous reaction, which we'll discuss further later in Part Two, is called the *myotatic reflex* or stretch reflex.

One might assume that when a muscle contracts that the feedback from the muscle spindle would stop. However, this is not the case, because it would create opportunity for the muscle to get injured. When a muscle is contracted, gamma motor neurons are activated, pulling slightly on the muscle spindle. This makes the muscle spindle send a message that the muscle is a little longer than it actually is. The purpose of this is purely to keep the alpha-gamma feedback loop active so that injury to the muscle does not occur.

Alpha and gamma motor neurons are activated by commands being sent from the brain and by automatic messages from the alpha-gamma loop. The brain sends messages telling the muscles to voluntarily contract, while the alpha-gamma loop automatically maintains the resting level of tension in the muscles. The sensory receptors of Ia axons adapt quickly, so when the extrafusal fibers of a muscle are chronically contracted, our proprioception adjusts so that we feel that the muscle is not as short or tight as it actually is. In other words, the increased level of contraction in our muscles actually begins to feel normal.

So as we sit at our computer day after day, our brain learns to keep us in a slouched posture by keeping certain muscles contracted, and our proprioceptive and vestibular systems allow us to get more and more comfortable in this unnatural position. Slouching forward begins to feel normal and even good, and sitting up straight takes effort and feels uncomfortable. We typically remain blissfully unaware of this subconscious adaptation until, one day, it finally causes us pain. The loss of sensory awareness that accompanies learned movement patterns is the final part of our discussion.

The word "awareness" has a New-Agey connotation which may cause people who are grounded in reality to think that it is a fictional concept made up by people tripping on acid. The truth is that awareness is an important and entirely real function of human consciousness. Awareness should be practiced and maintained, as it is critical to our personal safety, ability to have healthy interactions with other people, and of course, preventing ourselves from acquiring damaging motor patterns.

We can improve our awareness by focusing our conscious attention, a concept which is a bit more tangible. We can choose to focus our attention on any portion of the vast amount of sensory information coming into our brain. By focusing our eyes on one object, we are able to observe the tiniest details of the object while ignoring everything else in our visual field. By listening intently, we can hear a conversation happening at the next table in a noisy, crowded restaurant.

Likewise, we can focus our attention on our proprioceptive sensations. Let's use the simple example of tilting your head downward so as to look at the ground. This postural habit is becoming increasingly common among Americans due to constant use of smart phones and computers.

As you are reading these words, your head is likely tilted downward. Bring your eyes up from the page and look straight ahead, so that your head sits straight up and down on top of your spine. Notice how this position feels different than tilting your head downward. Also notice how quickly you return to the tilted downward position. Which position is more comfortable? Can you feel certain muscles that are contracted or released in each position? Can you find a way to relax your neck and shoulders while looking straight ahead?

Now that you have taken the time to notice the difference between what these two positions feel like, you will likely start to notice your head position more often. In fact, once you have noticed or learned something new it can be difficult to not notice it. This tendency of our brain to notice things we have just learned is referred to as the Baader-Meinhof phenomenon. If you haven't heard of it before, you probably will again soon.

You may have had the experience of learning a new word and then suddenly seeing that word everywhere. The Baader-Meinhof phenomenon is also known as the frequency illusion or recency effect, and it is a result of having focused your attention on something new. Once your conscious attention has been brought to this new word, or to an internal sensation such as the position of your head, you have become more aware of this new word or sensation. Each time you read that new word, you will consciously recognize it instead of subconsciously skimming over it. Likewise, now when you hold your head tilted forward, your brain will recognize that proprioceptive sensation rather than ignoring it.

You can think of attention as being focused and active, and awareness as being broad and relaxed. If you begin to pay attention to your proprioceptive sensations, you will become more aware of them; so with practice, you won't need to work so hard at noticing your body position and movement. It's like staying tuned in to a certain radio station so you can always hear it in the background.

As we gradually learn a posture or movement pattern, we get used to the proprioceptive sensations that accompany it, and we begin to notice them less and less. This loss of awareness makes it very easy to fall deeper and deeper into our learned patterns, and also makes it very difficult to change them. In order to improve our body mechanics, we need to have an accurate sense of our starting point. And unfortunately, unnatural and damaging movement patterns feel natural and correct because we have gradually adapted to them.

* * *

We've covered a great deal of information in this chapter, and I hope it is becoming clear how all of these processes work together. We are continuously sensing and moving, continuously learning new motor patterns and strengthening existing ones. We are constantly becoming more and less aware of various sensations in our body.

Most of us are born with the same innate ability and potential to sense, move and learn. Yet throughout the course of our lives, we each develop such unique motor patterns that it is hard to believe we all started in the same place. In the next chapter, we'll learn how our habitual motor patterns lead to muscle and joint pain, and how our patterns can actually damage the structure of our bodies.

CHAPTER 6

When Our Patterns Cause Pain

Our bodies do not break down for no reason, and age alone does not make physical degeneration inevitable. If it did, everyone over the age of eighty would be practically immobile, and people under the age of twenty would never suffer from any age-related degenerative conditions. Yet we see people close to a hundred years of age who continue to be active and pain-free, and teenagers with bulging discs, tendonitis, stress fractures and chronic pain.

We begin learning motor patterns as infants and the learning process continues throughout our entire lives. Somewhere along the way, the vast majority of us will experience some kind of pain or discomfort as a result of our learned motor patterns. The way we habitually stand and move is the main factor in how quickly and in what manner our bodies break down. In this chapter, we'll discuss how habitual motor patterns lead to many common musculoskeletal problems.

Muscle Spasms and Cramps

You may have a friend who throws his back out every few months and has to spend several days lying flat on his back in bed. Or maybe you are the unlucky one who has had to call for help getting up off the floor. Muscle spasms are no fun at all, and can be incapacitating when experienced in the back or neck.

Muscle spasms typically occur in muscles that are already being held chronically tight. In Part One we learned why tight muscles hurt: hydrogen ions that build up as a result of anaerobic metabolism activate nociceptors in the muscles, which are being held in a contraction. When people throw their backs out, it usually happens when they are doing something seemingly innocuous like reaching for a cup of coffee or bending over to brush their teeth. A small movement can put enough strain on the already tight back muscles that the stretch reflex is activated, causing the muscles to contract even more in order to prevent their fibers from tearing. Stay tuned—I'll explain the stretch reflex in detail in the next chapter.

A spasm can go on for many days, and typically the pain will gradually decrease as the muscles slowly release. We must go through a process of regaining voluntary control over the muscles that are being held involuntarily in spasm. One factor that can hinder this process is our natural tendency to hold painful parts of our body stiff. We do this subconsciously in order to effectively splint an injured body part and prevent further pain that might be caused by movement. Unfortunately, in the case of muscle spasms, we often increase our own pain by keeping the spasmodic muscles tight and preventing the movement that is necessary for us to regain voluntary control.

In contrast to spasms, muscle cramps are short-lived, intense involuntary contractions. Dehydration and electrolyte imbalance have traditionally been thought to be responsible for cramping. Many people may be surprised to find out that there is little evidence for this theory, and that research instead shows that repetitive muscular contraction, muscular fatigue, and the resulting loss of neuromuscular control are likely responsible for cramping. Cramping occurs most often in high-level athletes, and studies have found no electrolyte changes or body weight changes in these groups after performance. It is hypothesized that when muscle spindles get overexcited they can inhibit the activity of the Golgi tendon organ, reducing the relaxation phase of the muscle and causing it to go into a strong contraction.

Cramping can occur in non-athletes too. For example, many women who wear high heels often experience cramps in their calves and feet. Their calf and foot muscles are kept in a shortened, contracted state all day long, and by the end of the day the muscles are fatigued from the constant contraction.

So, how can you prevent muscle spasms and cramps? By reducing your resting level of muscle tension, relearning natural, efficient movement patterns, and allowing yourself time to rest when exercising.

Tendinitis

Tendons are a type of connective tissue which serve the important function of connecting muscles to bones. They are made up of densely packed collagen fibers arranged in parallel lines and a small amount of a protein called elastin, which allows tendons to return to their normal length after contracting or stretching.

When tendons are injured, inflammation will occur and cause pain; this is the condition of tendinitis. However, it has been found that most tendon pain is actually caused by chronic degeneration rather than acute inflammation. The suffix *-itis* refers to an acute condition, while the suffix *-osis* refers to a chronic condition. So, most tendon pain should actually be called tendinosis. In these cases, inflammation is not present, and the color of the tendon has turned from a healthy shiny white to a dull gray or brown. The tough collagen fibers have become soft and have begun to lose their ability to bear tension.

So if painful inflammatory substances aren't present, what causes the pain in tendinosis? Research shows that high levels of the amino acid glutamate are found in degenerating tendons, so it is likely that glutamate is at least partly responsible for the pain.

Dysfunctional movement patterns and general overuse are the main causes of tendinosis. Demanding too much of a tendon, or making it move in a way it is not designed to, will lead to the gradual breakdown and weakening of its collagen fibers.

Tendon pain, whether caused by inflammation or

degeneration, can be quite frustrating because it can take so long to subside. Tendons have limited blood supply, so the healing and rebuilding process can take much longer than that following an injury to muscle or skin. With time and patience, rest combined with retraining movement patterns will allow tendons to heal.

Plantar Fasciitis

The plantar fascia is a thick band of connective tissue which runs along the underside of the foot, from the heel bone to the metatarsal bones. Its function is to support the arch of the foot by carrying tension when the foot bears weight. When too much is demanded of the plantar fascia, either as a result of repetitive movements or constant strain from tight muscles or excessive body weight, the tissue can become inflamed and undergo degeneration.

Plantar fasciitis is most often experienced by runners and people who are overweight. But since only a portion of these folks ever feel plantar fasciitis pain, we know that overuse is only part of the problem. Habitual movement patterns involving tightness along the back of the legs and bottom of the feet are the other main contributing factor. Improper footwear, which I'll talk about in Part Four, can also be a culprit.

Bursitis

In every joint there are bursae, small sacs of connective tissue filled with synovial fluid, which look like little water balloons. They sit between bones and tendons, providing cushioning in the joint and allowing tendons to move easily over bone. When we overuse a joint, new bursae can actually grow in order to provide extra protection.

Bursitis occurs when a bursa gets inflamed and causes pain. When we repeat the same movement over and over, the tendon rubs against the bursa repeatedly, and after a while the bursa can become irritated. The inflammatory process increases the amount of fluid inside the bursa, and the increased pressure from the fluid causes pain. Muscles around the painful joint will often tighten up in order to splint the injury, limiting range of motion and compressing the joint—leading to more pain.

Adhesive Capsulitis

Every joint is protected by a joint capsule, a sleeve of dense connective tissue encasing cartilage and synovial fluid. In the condition of adhesive capsulitis, sometimes referred to as frozen shoulder, the joint capsule of the glenohumeral joint gradually becomes thicker and tighter, restricting the movement of the shoulder and causing pain.

Adhesive capsulitis seems to be directly related to lack of movement, as it often occurs in people who have undergone surgery or an injury in which they must keep their arm immobilized. Connective tissue adapts to the amount of movement demanded from it, becoming tighter with less movement and looser with more movement. This adaptation can lead to a vicious cycle: as connective tissues get tighter, movement becomes more difficult and sometimes painful, limiting movement further and allowing the tissues to tighten even more.

Temporomandibular Joint Disorders

The temporomandibular joint connects the jawbone to the skull, and is it one of the most complicated joints in the human body. It can open and close the jaw like a hinge, and allow the jaw to slide from side to side and forward and backward.

Temporomandibular joint (TMJ) disorders include many problems in and around the jaw, and these problems are most often caused by dysfunctional motor patterns and chronic muscle tension. The dysfunctional pattern causing the jaw pain is generally not limited to the jaw; many people with TMJ disorders have habitual patterns of muscular tension and pain in their neck and shoulders as well.

Stress is a major factor in developing tightness in and around the jaw. Stress causes us to clench our jaw and grind our teeth, even in our sleep. Learning to keep the jaw relaxed and identifying the sources of stress which trigger the pattern often allow TMJ issues to resolve swiftly.

Sciatica and Piriformis Syndrome

The sciatic nerve is the largest and thickest nerve in the human body. Nerves exiting the spine between the fourth lumbar vertebra and the third sacral vertebra come together to form the sciatic nerve, which runs through the buttocks and all the way down each leg. It is responsible for much of the sensory and motor innervation of the legs and feet. When the sciatic nerve is compressed you may feel shooting pain, a burning sensation, numbness or weakness in your legs and feet. Sciatica symptoms are generally caused when the nerves exiting the spine are compressed between the vertebrae by a bulging disc pressing against the nerve roots, or when the sciatic nerve is compressed after it has exited the spine.

In a small portion of the population, the sciatic nerve runs through a gluteal muscle called the piriformis instead of underneath it. For these people, chronic tightness in the piriformis can compress the sciatic nerve, causing piriformis syndrome. The symptoms of sciatica and piriformis syndrome are the same; the distinction is made based on where the nerve compression occurs.

Sciatica and piriformis syndrome are most often caused by habitual muscular tightness in the lower back and gluteal muscles, which leads to compression of the spine and the sciatic nerve. The symptoms typically clear up once the muscle tension is released and the dysfunctional movement patterns are retrained.

Thoracic Outlet Syndrome

Thoracic outlet syndrome is a condition in which the bundle of nerves and blood vessels responsible for sensation, motor control and circulation in the arm is compressed. The neurovascular bundle travels through the scalene muscles of the neck, between the collarbone and first rib (the area known as the thoracic outlet), under the pectoralis minor, and around the humerus. If the bundle is compressed at any point along its path, a person may feel shooting pain, numbness, weakness and tingling in the arm.

Chronic muscle tightness in the neck, chest and front of the shoulders leads to the compression that occurs in thoracic outlet syndrome. This syndrome most often occurs in people who must repeatedly contract these muscles, such as musicians, electricians, computer workers, and athletes like swimmers and baseball players. Thoracic outlet syndrome also occurs when people have experienced an injury such as a broken arm and must keep their arm in a sling for a long period of time; this leads to a tightening of the neck, chest and shoulders due to both lack of use and instinctive protecting of the injured area.

Carpal Tunnel Syndrome

The median nerve passes between the carpal bones of the wrist and the transverse carpal ligament, innervating portions of the forearm and hand. When this nerve is compressed, most often due to inflammation in the wrist joint and thickening of parts of the joint due to overuse, we experience carpal tunnel syndrome. This condition is characterized by shooting pain, burning, tingling, numbness and weakness in the hand. Carpal tunnel syndrome typically occurs in people who do repetitive tasks with their hands, such as computer workers, massage therapists and assembly line workers.

The joints of our extremities, such as the wrist joint, are designed to do less work than the joints closer to the center of our body. For example, in a reaching movement, most of the range of motion should come from a bending or twisting of the spine. Then the shoulder blade will slide to allow more movement, and lastly the joints of the arm and hand will articulate as needed in order to complete the task. People who experience carpal tunnel syndrome typically have chronic tension in their torso and shoulder, and have developed movement patterns in which they overuse their wrist joint and underuse the core of their body. They demand far more movement from their wrist than the joint is equipped to do, and irritation, inflammation and pain occur as a result.

Headache

Over forty-five million Americans suffer from chronic headaches. It is estimated that the cost of missed work and medical bills related to headaches total about fifty billion dollars per year. Headaches are among the most frustrating pain conditions because the causes are so varied. In fact, over a hundred and fifty different recognized types of headaches have been established by the International Classification of Headache Disorders.

There are no nociceptors in the brain tissue itself, so headaches are caused by pain felt in areas surrounding the brain: the head and neck muscles, blood vessels, eyes, ears, sinuses, and the membrane lining the outer surface of the skull. And despite an overwhelming list of possible causes, the odds are that your headache is due at least in part to muscular tension. Almost eighty percent of all headaches are classified as tension headaches, which can be brought on by habitual muscular contraction as well as stress, anxiety or injury. Tension headaches typically feel dull and aching, as if a band is tightening around your head.

The second most common type of headache is migraine,

which causes severe pain and often occurs along with vision changes or nausea. Migraine headaches can be hereditary, and so far two genes have been identified which are present in about half of migraine sufferers. It is believed that migraines are brought on when the trigeminal nerve, the largest of the cranial nerves, releases irritating chemicals that cause pain and swelling of blood vessels on the surface of the brain. Migraine pain is usually referred and felt in the eyes or temples. Migraines can be triggered by many controllable factors such as lack of sleep, certain foods, missing a meal, stress, caffeine withdrawal, alcohol and medications.

After muscle tension and migraine, there is a seemingly never-ending list of other causes of headaches: sinus pressure, viral infection, stress, premenstrual symptoms, stroke, high blood pressure, dehydration, caffeine withdrawal, alcohol consumption, allergies, celiac disease, heavy metal poisoning, carbon monoxide poisoning, and brain conditions such as infection, tumor and aneurysm. In addition, medication-overuse or "rebound" headaches can occur when people take pain medication more than three times per week. Yes, that's right—the exact medication which should be helping to relieve your headaches can actually be causing them.

If you suffer from chronic headaches, it will help both you and your doctor immensely if you begin to keep a headache journal. Spend a few weeks writing down everything you eat and drink, your sleep patterns, exercise habits, and sources of stress. Record everything about the headaches you experience: when they come on, how long they last, and what they feel like. Notice if relaxing activities, such as soaking in a hot tub or going on vacation, reduce your headache symptoms. If they do, stress and muscular tension are likely contributing to your headaches.

You will likely have to go through a process of experimentation and elimination to discover what factor or factors are causing your headaches. While it might take some time, it's worth it. Just because headaches are common, it doesn't mean you have to live with them.

When Function Changes Structure

Our bodies can only withstand so much. When a damaging movement pattern continues for a long period of time, our structure begins to break down. Constant compression, limited movement, and unnatural movement patterns cause soft tissues to tear, intervertebral discs to thin or rupture, cartilage in our joints to wear away, and stress fractures to form in otherwise healthy bones.

Spinal problems are among the most common issues resulting from dysfunctional movement habits. Made up of twenty-four articulating vertebrae, plus the fused sacral vertebrae and bones of the coccyx, the spine is a marvelous feat of engineering. It allows us to bend forward and backward, side to side, and twist in either direction. The vertebral column provides vital protection of our spinal cord while at the same bearing a great deal of weight and absorbing shock as we run, jump, and lift heavy objects.

The discs that sit in between each vertebra are quite strong and resilient. Each disc is made up of a tough outer layer of collagen fibers, called the annulus fibrosus, surrounding a soft core made of a gel-like substance, called the nucleus pulposus. The two structures work together to distribute pressure across the disc, providing essential cushioning between the vertebrae and allowing for bending and twisting, shock absorption, and weight bearing.

As we build up habitual muscle tension in our back, neck and entire trunk, increasing pressure is put on our spine, and our intervertebral discs suffer the consequences. The more the discs are compressed, the looser and weaker the fibers of the annulus fibrosus become. When compression is constant, a disc will begin to bulge or protrude out from its normal boundaries. Sometimes it will press on nerve roots or the spinal cord, causing pain or other nerve sensation. If the bulge doesn't press on nerve tissue, you may feel no pain or unusual sensation at all.

If a disc is put under a great deal of strain from constant compression or sudden increase in pressure it can rupture, allowing the contents of the nucleus pulposus to leak out. While this sounds like permanent damage, injured discs can be repaired if given the chance. The inflammatory process automatically kicks in to repair the disc, and if compression on the spine is reduced and motor patterns are improved, a ruptured disc can heal and resume its normal size and function.

Constant compression and imbalanced, unnatural movement patterns also affect the cartilage in joints throughout the body. Cartilage is a connective tissue that provides padding and protection in between bones. Most cartilage does not have a blood supply of its own, so it relies on the pumping action from joint movement to distribute blood and other nutrients via diffusion through joint fluid. Too much compression and too little compression both spell trouble for cartilage; it needs a moderate amount of movement, involving regular loading and unloading of weight, in order to remain healthy.

Our cartilage constantly maintains and rebuilds itself throughout our lives. However, cartilage grows and repairs itself fairly slowly due to the indirect way that it receives nutrients. If cartilage repair can't keep up with the rate at which we do damage, cartilage cells can completely wear away. The cells which produce new cartilage, called chondrocytes, are unable to migrate outside of their designated area; so once an area of cartilage is completely worn away, it's gone for good.

The painful condition of osteoarthritis is a result of a loss of healthy cartilage. Without the essential padding in between bones, our joints become quite stiff and painful. Reflexive tightening of the muscles surrounding the painful joints only worsens the condition by limiting range of motion. Osteoarthritis occurs most often as a result of the way we use our bodies, so in most cases it is preventable.

Dysfunctional movement patterns can go so far as to damage our bones. Bones rubbing together without the protection of cartilage can wear away, change shape, and develop growths called osteophytes. The way we move can even cause our bones to break. Repeated strain on a bone can cause a hairline fracture to form, and if the damaging movement continues, the stress fracture will continue to grow. Once a stress fracture is present, a sudden increase of pressure on the bone can be enough to break it completely.

There are times when it seems that we can't prevent the damage that is done to our bodies. Injuries can seem to come out of the blue, like when we strain a muscle, sprain an ankle, or dislocate a shoulder. But just as a chain will break at its weakest link, the parts of the body that are already compromised as a result of continuous dysfunction are the most likely areas to get injured when the body is under acute stress.

When muscles and tendons are stretched beyond their limit, their fibers will tear, causing what is known as a strain. A strong, unexpected force can cause a strain in any part of the body, but most often strains will occur in muscles and tendons that are tight due to habitual movement patterns.

Ligaments, the straps of connective tissue which connect bones to other bones, can also be torn. Both tendons and ligaments are made of collagen fibers, but ligaments have a more dense structure. As such, they provide less stretch and rebound than tendons and are more prone to tearing. Injuries to ligaments are called sprains, and they are generally more serious than muscle and tendon strains. Like tendons, ligaments have limited blood supply, so healing takes a long time. The structure of muscles and tendons allows them to regain their original length and strength after healing. In contrast, ligaments can become loose after being injured, making joints unstable and increasing the risk of dislocation and damage to cartilage.

Whiplash is one of the most common acute injuries that

results in chronic pain. Typically when whiplash occurs in a car accident, the head is first thrown backward and then forward. The sudden, extreme degree of movement can cause strains, sprains, and serious damage to the cervical vertebrae, discs, facet joints, temporomandibular joint, and spinal cord. And while this structural damage can be quite serious, the most common cause of long-term pain resulting from whiplash is muscle spasm. At the moment of impact, the neck muscles automatically contract in an attempt to stabilize the head while it is being thrown back and forth. After the injury, the muscles of the neck, and often the shoulders and back as well, will remain chronically contracted in order to splint the injury. This chronic contraction results in muscle pain and compression of the injured structure, potentially causing nerve pain, limiting blood flow, and slowing the healing process of injured discs and connective tissues.

* * *

If you have experienced any of the conditions we've covered in this chapter, you've likely been to your doctor, gotten a prescription for medication or physical therapy, and maybe visited a massage therapist or chiropractor as well. Most of the time, these approaches don't have much lasting effect because they don't address the underlying cause of the pain—the damaging motor pattern—which can only be changed through a process of active relearning. In the next chapter, we'll discuss the advantages and disadvantages of some of the most common pain treatments.

CHAPTER 7

Why Conventional Treatments Sometimes Work, but Often Don't

So, we've talked about how our learned motor patterns can lead to pain and actual damage to the structure of our body. The problem is coming from the inside: the way our nervous system is telling our body to stand and move. Knowing this, it would make sense to directly address our learned motor patterns when trying to treat musculoskeletal pain. Unfortunately, conventional pain treatments fail most of the time for two reasons. First, they approach pain as being a problem with the structure of the body rather than a problem with the functioning of the nervous system. Second, they focus on treating the area of the body where the pain is being felt instead of addressing the overall movement pattern that is causing pain and doing damage to the body.

Stretching

From a young age, we are taught that stretching is a necessary part of any workout routine. If we're involved in any type of athletics or physical training, we stretch to warm up, to cool down, and during breaks to help us stay loose. Unfortunately, stretching usually doesn't accomplish much, mainly due to the myotatic reflex, more commonly referred to as the stretch reflex.

Earlier in Part Two I described how the stretch reflex works. Here's a refresher: When a muscle is stretched, the sensory axons wrapped around the muscle spindle sense the increase in length and send this information to the alpha motor neuron in the spine. The alpha motor neuron then immediately sends the message to the extrafusal muscle fibers to contract in order to protect the muscle from being torn. The neurons carrying these messages back and forth from the spine are among the most heavily myelinated in the body; this means that their messages travel faster and are more important to our survival than the sensations of pain, touch and temperature.

One critical function of the stretch reflex is that it helps us stand up straight in our gravitational field. For example, when a person standing upright begins to lean to the right side, the postural muscles on the left side of the vertebral column will be stretched. When the muscle spindles in those muscles sense that they are being lengthened, they automatically send the message to contract in order to correct the person's posture. We are rarely consciously aware of how the stretch reflex automatically maintains our balance and keeps us from falling over—but we sure would notice if it wasn't working properly.

The stretch reflex also exists to prevent us from tearing our muscles, tendons and ligaments. The knee-jerk reflex is a great example. The doctor hits your patellar tendon just below your knee, suddenly stretching the tendon and the quadriceps muscle to which it is attached. The muscle spindles in your quadriceps senses the sudden increase in length and automatically sends the message to contract your quadriceps in order to prevent injury and over-stretching of the muscle and tendon. When your quadriceps contracts, your foot kicks up. If your foot doesn't kick up, it could be a potential sign of a neurological disorder, such as receptor damage or peripheral nerve disease.

When you practice static stretching (the type of stretching traditionally taught in athletic training), the conscious and sub-conscious parts of your nervous system are battling against each other, trying to achieve opposite results. The conscious part of your brain is sending the message to manually stretch your muscles by pulling on them. But despite all your efforts, your stretch reflex is automatically kicking in, contracting your muscles to prevent you from overstretching and tearing your muscles, tendons and ligaments.

So if our stretch reflex prevents us from manually lengthening our muscles, why does stretching sometimes make us more flexible? There are a few reasons. One is that when you engage in prolonged static stretching, pulling your muscles and tendons past the point that they are able to voluntarily lengthen, you begin to stretch your ligaments. We learned in the last chapter that ligaments have little ability to rebound the way muscles and tendons do. With prolonged stretching, ligaments can be stretched, resulting in more flexible and often less stable joints. Once stretched, ligaments may never regain their original length and strength.

Second, prolonged static stretching can cause the stretch reflex to become much less active, leaving the muscles lengthened for a period of time. This is why you may feel looser after you stretch, but unfortunately, the effects wear off fairly quickly. Often you will feel your muscles begin to tighten up again within just a few hours as your stretch reflex regains normal function.

For this reason, prolonged static stretching also decreases muscle performance by temporarily reducing the muscle's ability to contract. This is no good if you're about to play an important game. A great deal of research has shown that static stretching before a workout decreases joint stability and reduces muscle performance, strength and power. Many coaches and trainers have come to realize that the best way to warm up is to do a slow, gentle version of the movement you'll be doing in your workout. By consciously practicing the movement sequences and increasing blood flow to your muscles and connective tissues, this type of warm up prepares both your brain and your body for optimal performance.

The third reason why stretching can make us feel more flexible is that when we stretch repeatedly, we are building up a tolerance to the sensation of pulling in our muscles.

Even though it is by nature an uncomfortable sensation, with repetition it can become tolerable and even enjoyable. As a ballet dancer, I loved that feeling of pulling on my muscles and I craved it every day. It provided me with a temporary lengthening and release of my muscles, and as I became more comfortable with the feeling, I was able to pull my muscles even farther. But of course the reason I craved that feeling every day is that the fix was only temporary. Less than twenty-four hours after stretching, my muscles had tightened right back up again.

Virtually everyone I meet who has tried stretching to relieve their chronic pain reports that it hasn't helped them at all, and there are two simple reasons why. First, stretching does not reeducate the nervous system. No amount of pulling on the muscles will change the resting level of muscle tension that is being set by the alpha-gamma loop. This must be reset through an active process of relearning involving slow, conscious, voluntary movement and the integration of sensory feedback from the muscle.

Second, when you pull on an already tight muscle the stretch reflex is activated, making the muscle contract even more. It is possible that you might find some relief from gentle prolonged stretching, but as we've already discussed, the increased muscle length is temporary and the muscle will rebound within a short period of time. Most likely, stretching will not only do little for your pain, but will likely increase and prolong your pain by making your muscles tighter.

When I finally stopped stretching and started exclusively practicing the techniques I'll discuss in Parts Three and Four,

I felt like I had a brand-new body. Instead of feeling tight and uncomfortable all the time, I began to feel loose, comfortable and completely relaxed.

Massage

If you've had a massage lately, you may have found yourself faced with a never ending list of different varieties, including acupressure, Ayurvedic, deep tissue, hot stone, lymphatic, Shiatsu, sports and Thai. Massage therapy has become overwhelmingly popular, and rightfully so; in addition to feeling good, it has a number of health benefits.

Massage therapy uses various techniques to apply pressure on muscles and connective tissues in order to lengthen tissues, relieve pain, relax the nervous system, and stimulate the circulatory system. Hippocrates defined it simply as "the art of rubbing." It is one of the oldest types of physical therapy, appearing in written records from several thousand years ago and likely predating recorded history. Massage was developed in eastern and middle-eastern cultures, and gained popularity in Europe during the Renaissance. In the second half of the nineteenth century, Dutch massage therapist Johan Georg Mezger named the basic massage strokes and codified them in a method which we know today as Swedish massage or classic massage.

So, why is massage so popular? Mainly because it feels good, especially if we're in pain. Here's why: the nerves that carry information about the sensation of touch to the brain are more heavily myelinated than the nerves which carry information about pain. So, touch information travels faster than pain information. This is why we instinctively rub the skin around a painful area; the touch sensation temporarily drowns out the pain sensation, and we are given a brief moment of relief.

Massage also feels good because it temporarily reduces muscle tension. Pressing on tight muscles lengthens them in the same way that gentle prolonged static stretching does, and after an hour or so of this manual lengthening you may stand up feeling like your muscles are made of jelly. Unfortunately, within a few hours you will likely experience what one of my clients called the "rebound effect." Your muscles begin to tighten up again as your stretch reflex regains normal function, and by the next day you'll back to your original level of tension.

If your massage therapist applies a great deal of pressure, your stretch reflex may get activated right away and you may wind up feeling tight and sore soon after a massage. A good rule of thumb is that if you feel pain during a massage, you're probably going to feel some soreness afterward as well. While it can be difficult in the moment, because you're so relaxed or don't want to offend, it is better to ask your massage therapist to press more gently than to have to suffer the consequences later. It is absolutely not necessary to apply a painful amount of pressure in order to reap the benefits of a massage. Moreover, if you're in pain a deep massage can increase and prolong your pain by making your muscles tighter.

Besides feeling good, another benefit of massage is that it softens connective tissues. But again, this effect is temporary. Tendons, ligaments, fascia (which surrounds, supports and separates structures of the body), and scar tissue (which forms to heal an injury) are all made of collagen fibers, arranged in varying patterns and densities. As muscles become habitually tighter and movement decreases, connective tissues respond by getting tighter. Movement and heat have the effect of making these collagen structures more flexible and fluid.

It came as a surprise to the massage community when research came out showing that myofascial release techniques have little to no lasting effect on fascia. The results of the research showed that fascia does not respond to manual stretching because it is not simply a collagen structure—it actually contains smooth muscle cells, and is innervated by four different types of mechanoreceptors. Thus, the best way to make fascia more loose and flexible is by reeducating the nervous system through active movement.

In addition to its temporary effects on the physical structure of our body, massage affects our functioning by cueing the nervous system to relax. One study showed that a single session of Swedish massage significantly decreased the release of both the stress hormone cortisol and the hormone arginine vasopressin, which raises blood pressure and constricts blood vessels. Massage also stimulates the circulatory system and lymphatic system, improving blood flow and elimination of wastes in the body.

Most significantly, massage provides the sensation of touch, which is critical in both early childhood development and our overall health as adults. Two fairly shocking reports in 1915 revealed that at least ninety percent of infants in

American orphanages died within one year of admission even though they had received adequate physical care. The few infants who survived suffered severe physical and mental retardation. As it turned out, the missing element in the infants' care was tactile stimulation. When the orphanages brought on additional staff, each infant was held and played with every day, and mortality rates fell dramatically.

Levels of the hormone somatotrophin, known as "human growth hormone," have been found to correlate directly with the amount of physical contact we receive. As children, we need a great deal of growth hormone in order to fully develop. We need less of this hormone as adults, but the small amount that we do need is critical for cellular healing and growth. Tactile stimulation affects the immune system as well; a study of breast cancer patients showed that regular massages improved the patients' immune response. Research also suggests the benefits of touch for a variety of conditions such as anxiety, autism, ADHD, cardiovascular disease, Alzheimer's disease, depression, aggressive behavior, stroke, and sleep disturbances.

The benefits of massage for chronic pain do exist, but as we have already discussed, they are temporary. Massage alone is very rarely enough to change deeply learned movement habits or the habituated resting level of muscle tension. The sensory education and awareness that can be gained through massage is valuable, but if it is not followed up by actual motor education in the form of voluntary movement, little lasting progress will be made.

Chiropractic

Ancient Chinese and Greek cultures understood how vital the spine is to our functioning, and they practiced techniques of spinal manipulation to ease back pain and improve health. Spinal manipulation began gaining popularity in the United States in the late nineteenth century when Daniel David Palmer founded the Palmer School of Chiropractic in Iowa.

The practice of chiropractics is based on the idea that joints become either restricted or hypermobile due to soft tissue injury caused by acute trauma or repetitive stresses. Chiropractic care is focused heavily on working with the spine and correcting vertebral subluxations, which occur when individual vertebrae become displaced or dysfunctional. Doctors of chiropractic work with a variety of musculoskeletal conditions, such as back and neck pain, bulging or herniated discs, headaches, whiplash, nerve sensation and pain, and other chronic pain conditions such as fibromyalgia.

When chiropractors perform spinal manipulations, often referred to as chiropractic adjustments, they apply controlled force into a joint which moves the joint back into proper alignment. Adjustments are typically performed quickly and require patients to remain fully relaxed so that they do not resist the movement. It is believed that bringing joints back into alignment restores mobility, alleviates muscle tightness and pain, and allows injuries to heal.

Chiropractic adjustments, or any movements which pop a joint back into alignment, usually provide an enjoyable sense of release and relief from pressure or pain. Unfortunately—

and if you've been paying attention so far, you know what I'm about to say—the fact is that simply manipulating the structure of the body does not change the way it is functioning. Within a few days or even just a few hours of an adjustment, your learned movement patterns and habituated level of muscle tension will typically cause your joints to become misaligned again, and you'll be making an appointment for another adjustment.

A number of studies have shown a lack of evidence for the effectiveness of spinal adjustments for back pain. Of greater concern is the risk of increased or radiating pain, headaches, and dizziness following an adjustment. Case studies have also reported instances of more serious adverse effects such as stroke, disc herniation, spinal cord injury, and epidural hematoma. When going through chiropractic treatment you should be aware of the risks involved, and should also keep a journal noting how you feel each day. If your condition is not improving, pursuing chiropractic care is probably not worth the potential adverse effects.

The Bottom Line

While the techniques we've discussed so far in this chapter have some benefits, none of them address the underlying cause of pain, structural misalignment, and physical degeneration. Our bones do not move unless our muscles make them move, and our muscles do not move unless directed to by our nervous system. It is the functioning of our nervous system which determines how we move, what type of pain we experience, and ultimately how much damage we do to our bodies. The bottom line is that voluntary movement is necessary in order to reeducate the nervous system and change habitual motor patterns. On that note, let's talk about the only mainstream treatment for musculoskeletal pain that is based on voluntary movement: physical therapy.

Physical Therapy

While many physical therapists employ massage and other passive manipulation techniques, the focus of physical therapy is on the regular practice of active movements in order to improve function, reduce pain, and recover from injury. Pehr Henrik Ling, who developed medical-gymnastics and contributed to the development of massage in Western cultures, was also fundamental in establishing physical exercise as an acceptable way to treat pain and illness. During the late nineteenth and early twentieth centuries, various forms of physical therapy became quite popular and professional schools were established. The polio epidemic in the United States during the 1940s and 1950s created great demand for physical therapists, and the profession grew exponentially.

Research provides clear evidence for the efficacy of physical therapy, not only for recovery from acute injury but also for chronic pain conditions. When people with back pain go through physical therapy treatment involving active exercises, they experience greater reductions in pain, more improvements in function, use less medication, and have lower health care costs than people who receive passive therapy treatments. Research also shows that the earlier someone has physical therapy, the better. The longer the pain condition goes on, the higher their health care costs and the more likely they are to require injections or surgery.

A physical therapist may prescribe exercises which are designed to improve strength, range of motion, mobility, and balance, depending on the needs of the patient. Strength-building exercises are typically focused on the site of the injury; so a person recovering from shoulder surgery will be taught exercises to build up strength in the muscles around the shoulder joint. This approach can be very effective in building strength and regaining function after an injury or surgery. However, it still doesn't address the full body pattern that likely contributed to the injury or degeneration in the first place.

While there are many benefits to physical therapy, there are two main reasons why chronic pain patients might not have success with it. First is that strength-building exercises are typically prescribed in order to fix imbalances in posture and movement. Lack of strength is typically not the issue for people in chronic pain. Most often, it is chronic tightness and damaging movement patterns. Strength-building exercises can result in making the targeted muscles tighter, which can increase muscle soreness and pain. What people in chronic pain most often need is for chronically tight muscles to be released, not strengthened.

The second reason why physical therapy may not work for people in chronic pain is that it does not address full-body movement patterns. For example, let's say a man has pain in his left knee. He most likely is standing and moving in such a way that undue pressure is being put on his knee, and muscles and connective tissues around the knee are pulling and pushing on the joint in unnatural ways. All of this pressure and imbalance is creating inflammation and pain, and over time will lead to degeneration of the joint. Strength-building exercises focusing on the knee will likely not help him at this point; the way he is moving his entire body needs to be addressed.

If this man gets to the point at which some or all the cartilage in his knee has been worn away, he will likely have a knee replacement or a cartilage transplant. Either of these surgeries will most likely help him a great deal in the short term by reducing his pain. However, if the movement pattern which caused the damage in the first place is not addressed, further damage can occur. He may experience loss of the new cartilage, pain in his knee or another area of his body, or the need for a second joint replacement.

Medication

When you're in pain, any relief from the constant aching, throbbing or burning can feel like a miracle. Relief provided by pain medication, however brief, can have profound positive effects on our mental and emotional state. Most importantly, when used appropriately in acute pain conditions such as injury and surgery, pain medication can actually prevent future chronic pain from developing.

We've already learned about how neuroplastic changes occur in the nervous system when pain is experienced for a long period of time. The nervous system can become sensitized, and the sensation of pain can remain or increase even if the source of the pain has healed. We learned in Part One how strategic use of medication to block pain early on, such as before surgery, can prevent this sensitization from occurring. Medication can also be given during surgery for the same effect. This technique has been proven to have positive results in preventing the development of chronic pain after surgery. Considering that up to three-quarters of surgical patients develop chronic pain conditions, use of medication before or during surgery seems to be an approach that should be used as often as possible in an effort to reduce the risk of chronic pain.

Pain medications work in various ways to block the sensation of pain. Non-opioid analgesics, the most common of which are acetaminophen and ibuprofin, work by blocking the production of prostaglandins, a group of lipid compounds which play a role in fever, inflammation and pain. Acetaminophen prevents the production of prostaglandins in the central nervous system, while ibuprofin blocks the production throughout the body. This is why ibuprofin can reduce inflammation at the site of an injury while acetaminophen can't, and why ibuprofin can irritate the lining of the stomach and cause liver and kidney damage while acetaminophen won't.

Another type of non-opioid analgesic drugs are corticosteroids, powerful anti-inflammatories that can be taken orally or injected. Cortisone is produced naturally by the adrenal gland and released into the bloodstream when the body is under stress. Injectable cortisone is a synthetic version of our natural cortisone, and is injected directly into the joint or soft tissue where inflammation is occurring. Cortisone has become popular among athletes and non-athletes alike.

While cortisone injections can be quite effective in providing temporary pain relief, research has shown that they are counterproductive to long-term recovery. Pain patients who receive injections have a lower rate of recovery than patients who undergo physical therapy or do nothing at all. And patients who get injections are sixty-three percent more likely to experience a relapse of their injury compared to people who have no treatment. Predictably, the more injections a patient receives, the lower chance they have of full recovery. Injections also pose serious short-term risks including infection, increased pain, softening of cartilage, and weakening or rupture of tendons.

In Part One we discussed opioids and how they block the sensation of pain by binding to opioid receptors. Like all pain medications, their effect is only temporary, and opioids pose the added risk of dependence and addiction. The nervous system can become dependent upon opioids within just a week of regular use, and tolerance develops quickly, requiring the patient to take higher doses to get the same level of pain relief. Opioids can also have dangerous side effects when mixed with alcohol and some antidepressants, antihistamines, and sleeping pills. Due to the associated risks, opioids are best used for short periods of time in conditions of acute pain when their dosage can be monitored by a health care professional.

Another risk of pain medication, which is of utmost concern to me, is that masking pain with drugs gives us the opportunity to do further damage to our bodies. Athletes get cortisone shots and then resume playing; this only serves to make their injury worse, lengthen their recovery time, and increase their chances of needing surgery. Non-athletes take their daily dose of ibuprofin or prescribed opioid and then go about their daily lives, continuing to engage in the activities and movement habits which caused their pain or injury in the first place. Pain medication allows people to prolong and sometimes worsen their condition, and gives them the misconception that they have found a solution. Since many people can relieve and even eliminate their pain through re-education of the nervous system, simply managing pain with medication is not an acceptable solution.

Surgery

We talked about the dangers of surgery and its lack of effectiveness for chronic pain conditions in the first chapter of the book. I'd like to round out that discussion here by making a couple of brief points.

First, there are cases of chronic pain for which surgery is absolutely the best course of treatment. When the structure of the body is damaged to the point that it cannot repair itself with rest and improved movement, surgery is probably the way to go. Joint replacement surgeries in particular have become highly successful. But remember that surgery will not change your learned movement patterns. These patterns will still be present after the surgery and will likely continue to do damage to your body, potentially demanding repeat surgeries. Surgeries to repair chronic musculoskeletal pain and degeneration should always be followed up with movement re-education in order to address the original underlying cause of the condition.

Second, there are some surgical techniques that target pain perception by working with or altering the nervous system. Electrical stimulators can be implanted near the spine to help manage and reduce pain. Surgeons can destroy portions of peripheral nerves, and can even sever pain pathways in the spinal cord and brain. These options should only be considered for cases of extreme chronic pain which have not improved with other treatments. And if pain perception really is the issue, it is possible that the pain could be reduced or even eliminated by re-educating the nervous system.

* * *

Usually by the time people come to me for lessons they have tried every possible treatment for their pain. Some of the approaches have improved their condition for a period of time, but most have not helped at all. This is because no amount of external force, manipulation, drugs or surgery will change the automatic, subconscious messages being sent by your brain.

Thankfully, over the past hundred years or so, some curious, brilliant people figured this out. During the twentieth century, a series of movement educators and scientists began to explore the ways in which the habitual use of our body affects our health and functioning. In the next chapter, you'll read their stories and find out what they discovered.

PART THREE
SOLVING THE MYSTERY

CHAPTER 8

A Century of Exploration

The great phase in man's advancement is that in which he passes from subconscious to conscious control of his own mind and body.

F.M. ALEXANDER

Frederick Matthias Alexander was a precocious child. Born in 1869, he was the eldest child in large family. Growing up on a farm in Tasmania, Australia, he learned the value of self-sufficiency and problem solving at a young age. His energetic and attention-seeking nature led him to be taken out of school and taught privately. His teacher introduced him to the work of Shakespeare and ignited his lifelong love of the theater; he loved reading the plays aloud and interpreting the characters. Unfortunately, he suffered from health problems which included respiratory difficulties, so reciting and performing were often challenging.

At the age of sixteen, Alexander was offered a job at a tin-mining company in Mount Bischoff. Financial pressures forced him to take the position, and he worked diligently during the daytime while pursuing training in drama and music at night. After three years, Alexander had saved up a great deal of money, and he decided to move to Melbourne to pursue a career as an actor and reciter.

After reciting professionally for a number of years, Alexander's ongoing respiratory problems began to interfere with his work. Friends in the audience could hear him gasping for air as he spoke and he would occasionally become hoarse during performances. Upon visiting a doctor, Alexander was diagnosed with irritation of the mucous membrane of the throat and inflammation of the vocal chords. He was advised to have surgery to shorten his uvula, but he declined.

After resting his voice for two weeks, Alexander took the stage for an important performance. His doctor had assured him that after this period of rest his throat and vocal chords would be back to normal. Sadly, less than halfway through the performance Alexander's voice began to fail, and by the end of the evening he could barely speak.

Since rest had not helped, and since his hoarseness occurred only during performances and not during normal conversation, Alexander concluded that there had to be something he was doing during performances—something about the way he was using his voice—that was causing him to lose function of his vocal chords. Ever the problem-solver, he set about to figure out what it was.

Alexander knew that whatever it was he was doing, he was doing it subconsciously, so he would need a third-person perspective to give him an accurate assessment. He decided to observe himself in a mirror while speaking conversationally and while reciting. He noticed that as soon as he started reciting he would habitually pull his head back, compressing his larynx and causing him to gasp audibly as he breathed. Upon closer observation, Alexander noticed that these same habits were present during his normal speech, though to a much lesser extent.

Alexander hypothesized that the way he was unconsciously moving and holding himself while reciting was directly causing his vocal problems. He wondered if one habit caused the others. Was his improper breathing the culprit? Or was it the way he habitually pulled his head back, or the compressing of his larynx that was causing his voice to fail?

After months of experimenting, Alexander found that he was able to prevent himself to some degree from pulling his head back while reciting. This adjustment led to an improvement in his other two habits. As Alexander gradually changed his deeply learned patterns, he began to regain full use of his voice, and his tendency to become hoarse decreased. Doctors examined him and confirmed that the condition of his throat and vocal chords had improved considerably. Alexander's hypothesis was confirmed: the way he was using his body had directly affected the way he was functioning.

Alexander experimented extensively with holding his head and neck in different positions as he spoke, trying to find a way to optimize the use of his voice. Over time, he realized that how he moved his head and neck directly affected the way he used his entire torso. He observed that any misuse of his head and neck caused his posture to become unnatural and his stature to shorten. This observation was an incredibly important discovery for him. Alexander began to understand the larger patterns of tension involving his head, neck and torso, and that the use of one part directly affected the use of the others. He later termed this relationship of the head, neck and torso "Primary Control."

As Alexander continued to explore, he made more discoveries. Though he felt that he was making a great deal of progress in retraining himself, he noticed that when he performed for an audience he still had the tendency to automatically go into his old habits; the stress of performing always triggered his familiar movement patterns. He decided to experiment with what he called "inhibition." He practiced not responding at all to the stimulus of performing. By becoming comfortable with not automatically reacting when under the pressure of a performance, he was able to begin inhibiting his old patterns of misuse.

Alexander realized that focusing on the end goal of performing had been causing him to rely on habitual patterns. By slowing down and consciously concentrating on how he was reacting, he was able to teach himself to react differently. Alexander called this approach "means whereby." By focusing on the means whereby he was achieving the goal rather than on the goal itself, he was able to change the way that he accomplished the goal. By focusing on his process, his end result was much improved.

The endless hours he spent in front of a mirror provided Alexander with another critical insight. He became aware that his internal sense of how he was using his body was quite different than what he saw in the mirror. He also observed that standing and moving in a way that he knew intellectually to be correct often felt wrong and unnatural. He was experiencing firsthand how our proprioceptive senses adjust as our motor patterns become habitual. The mirror proved to be an invaluable tool in Alexander's exploration; had he relied purely on his internal sense of how he was using his body, he would have made little progress.

As Alexander's voice improved he became quite well known in Melbourne, and many actors sought him out for vocal coaching. Local doctors heard about his success in working with functional disorders and began referring patients to him. Alexander soon had a busy practice, with the majority of his students coming to him for treatment of medical conditions rather than vocal coaching.

As Alexander began to use his methods to work with others, he found that their proprioceptive senses were often inaccurate, just as his had been. Later in his career, after many years of teaching students, he concluded that "the prevalence of sensory untrustworthiness is of the utmost significance in relation to the problem of the control of human reaction." As he and his students experienced, with continued practice and retraining the proprioceptive senses could become trustworthy again.

In 1904, Alexander was convinced to move to London by

the surgeon J.W. Steward McKay, who wanted Alexander's work to get the recognition that it deserved. Alexander's practice in London flourished until the beginning of World War I, when he was forced to begin traveling back and forth from London to New York in order to stay busy. Demand for his work grew on both continents, and after years of people asking him to teach his methods, he launched a three-year teacher training course in 1931. Many doctors applied to the training, having witnessed the effects of Alexander's techniques in both themselves and their patients.

While Alexander had predominantly worked with adults for many years, he had a great love of working with children. As knowledge of his work spread, parents began sending their children to him to work with conditions of nervousness, inability to concentrate, speech difficulties, learning disabilities, flat feet, and rounded shoulders. With the help of teacher Irene Tasker and others, Alexander established the "little school," a division of his school which was devoted to teaching children. He strongly believed that his work should be utilized as education rather than re-education—that learning proper use of the self early in life would prevent more serious functional disorders later in life.

When Alexander first began his explorations, he believed that all illnesses or deficiencies were either mental or physical in nature. Over time, he realized that the mind and body are inextricably linked and while one may predominate, every human process and condition involves both the mind and body. Since the function of all parts of the human organism are connected, change in one part will affect the whole, and any attempt to create change must work with the whole person in order to be successful.

Alexander was among the first to recognize that voluntary human functioning is the cause of a myriad of health problems. His work marked the beginning of what would come to be known as "somatic education," a general term that describes methods of education which improve physiological function by increasing sensory-motor awareness and changing habitual patterns.

Alexander, known to his students as F.M., passed away in 1955 at the age of 86. His work continues to be taught in professional training programs that are held both in London and internationally, and there are more than 2,500 registered teachers of the Alexander Technique practicing worldwide. The method of education that Alexander developed inspired and contributed to the work of many other pioneers in the field of somatic education.

Elsa Gindler

Elsa Gindler was born in 1885 to a working class family in Berlin, Germany. As a young woman she suffered from consumption, known today as tuberculosis. Her doctor recommended a period of rest in Switzerland during which her affected lung could heal. Gindler could not afford such an expensive treatment, so she decided to try to rest her infected lung by using only her healthy lung to breathe. By paying close attention to her internal sensations, she gradually gained control of all the muscles involved in breathing into each lung independently.

As Gindler's health improved, her doctor called it a miracle, refusing to believe that such self-healing was possible. Like Alexander, Gindler had healed herself by focusing her attention inward and teaching herself to gain control of her physiological functioning.

Gindler became a physical education teacher, teaching a technique developed by Hedwig Kallmeyer called Harmonische Gymnastik. After some years of teaching this method she began to find it limiting, and she started to explore how to guide people through independent exploration of their sensory awareness. She stopped using the word "exercise" and began calling her movements "experiments."

Gindler asked her students to focus their attention completely on their internal sensations as they moved. She understood the principles of attention and awareness, in that the more conscious attention we pay to a part of our body, the greater sensation and motor control we develop. As their sensory awareness and motor control improved, Gindler's students experienced profound changes in their health and functioning.

Around 1924, Gindler met Heinrich Jacoby, a musician and educator who had a passion for psychoanalysis. The two studied together and collaborated on work which combined sensory exploration and psychotherapy. Sadly, they were forced to part ways when the Nazi regime took power in 1933. Jacoby left Germany for Switzerland, where he continued his work. Gindler stayed in Berlin, teaching her methods and providing shelter to those who were being persecuted for being of the Jewish faith.

Gindler did not wish to offer professional training in her methods; she simply wanted to do research and lead people through explorations in small study groups. Luckily, Gindler's students traveled and spread knowledge of her work. Most notably, her student Charlotte Selver emigrated to the United States and introduced Gindler's work under the name "Sensory Awareness." Selver and Gindler's other students influenced the work of many somatic educators and psychotherapists, including Erich Fromm, Fritz Perls, Alan Watts, Marion Rosen, Mary Wigman, Peter Levine and Wilhelm Reich.

Gerda Alexander

Gerda Alexander, of no relation to F.M., was born in 1908 in Wuppertal, Germany, to parents who had a love of music and movement. She began dancing as soon as she could stand. As she grew older, she studied the work of Emile Jacques-Dalcroze, called Eurhythmics, a method which taught students about music and dance by focusing on internal sensations rather than imitation of movement.

As a young woman, Alexander suffered from rheumatic fever and heart disease. Doctors told her that her dancing career was over and that she would spend the rest of her life in a wheelchair. Forced to rest for long periods of time, Alexander taught herself how to regulate her muscle tone and move with as little effort as possible so as not to strain her heart. Gradually, her health improved and in time she completely recovered. Contrary to her doctor's prognosis, she was able to dance again and began teaching Eurhythmics as well.

In 1929, as the Great Depression wrought worldwide havoc and the German government began to collapse, Alexander moved to Copenhagen, Denmark. There she began exploring ways to guide others through sensory experiments and movements which would allow them to improve their health and functioning. In 1940, she established a professional training school where she instructed students in her technique of "Eutony," a term derived from the Greek words for "good" and "tension."

Alexander spent the rest of her life dedicated to the exploration of human sensation and movement. She traveled around Europe, to Israel, and to North and South America, giving lectures about her research and methods to groups of dancers, movement therapists and psychotherapists.

Moshe Feldenkrais

Moshe Feldenkrais was born in 1904 to a Jewish family living in the small town of Slavuta, Russia. He developed a passion for math and physics at a young age, and the burgeoning fields of neurology and psychology intrigued him. By the age of twelve he was reading the works of Swiss psychotherapist and biologist August Forel.

At fourteen, Feldenkrais moved to Palestine to help build a Zionist society. There he worked and finished school, and became involved with Jewish defense groups, which introduced him to the martial art of jujitsu. Spending time with these groups sparked a passion for self-defense that would last his entire life. In particular, Feldenkrais became interested in unarmed defensive techniques in which one uses the body in a natural way to defend oneself without a great deal of physical effort. Wanting to develop a way by which people could learn how to effectively defend themselves, he conducted a study about how people respond to sudden attack and published a book on the topic in 1930.

That same year, Feldenkrais moved to Paris to study engineering. Upon graduating he began working as a research assistant in the laboratory of Frederic Joliot-Curie, son-in-law of Pierre and Marie Curie. During this time he met Jigaro Kano, the founder of modern judo. Inspired by Kano, Feldenkrais became Europe's first black belt Judoka in 1936. He stayed in Paris until 1940, working with nuclear fission in the lab and studying and teaching Judo.

Feldenkrais fled to England when the Germans invaded Paris in 1940. He continued his scientific work as an officer in the British Admiralty, developing radar for anti-submarine warfare in Scotland for five years. While in Scotland he taught Judo and self-defense classes, and published a self-defense manual titled *Practical Unarmed Combat*. The cover showed a soldier lying on his back on the ground, holding his machine gun in the air as if to surrender to the unarmed soldier who is easily overpowering him.

Feldenkrais had suffered an injury to his left knee during a soccer match in 1929, and had injured his right knee while working on a submarine in Scotland. He refused surgery even though the cruciate ligaments were damaged. Feldenkrais approached his knee injuries as an engineering problem, experimenting with moving and using his body in ways that would not put undue force on his knees. While working with the Admiralty, he began to give lectures and teach movement classes in his experimental methods.

After the war, Feldenkrais moved to London, where he delved into research on all areas of human functioning. He studied the work of F.M. Alexander, Elsa Gindler, Gerda Alexander, American physician William Bates, and Russian philosopher George Gurdjieff. In 1949, he published his first book on his own method of sensory-motor education, titled *Body and Mature Behavior*. The following year he traveled to Switzerland to work privately with Heinrich Jacoby, whom he greatly respected. The two men met ten times during June of 1950 to exchange ideas on learning and human potential. Feldenkrais considered their meetings to be exceptional learning experiences.

Feldenkrais's predecessors had relied mainly on experience-based research to develop their methods of sensory-motor education. Feldenkrais strove to combine science and experience, and did a great deal of research into human development, learning, and the functioning of the nervous system. He was able to see that at that point in time, scientists understood "so little about the functioning of the nervous system as a complete unit, that we have little right to expect any theory to be near the truth."

Yet Feldenkrais strove to develop a theory which would explain the dysfunction and physical degeneration he saw in his students and himself. He was especially interested in the way that humans move within gravity and the functioning of anti-gravity reflexes. He understood how our vestibular system allows us to constantly sense where we are in relation to gravity and how our automatic reflexes allow us to easily stand upright. He observed that many adults develop learned motor patterns which overpower their reflexive responses, resulting in maladaptive postural patterns that put a great deal of strain on the body.

Feldenkrais's experience in engineering and physics gave him a unique perspective on human functioning. He observed that the structure of the human body, with a high center of gravity balancing on two thin legs and two relatively small bases of the feet, was ideally suited for movement rather than static standing, which requires a heavy, broad base. Standing perfectly upright with all parts stacked vertically is fairly effortless for humans, but a great deal of effort is required to maintain any posture in which our center of gravity is not directly on top of our base. Since our reactions to gravity are almost always subconscious—because they are either reflexive or habitual—Feldenkrais knew that gravity must be taken out of the picture in order for unlearning of these involuntary patterns to occur. In order to prevent the automatic triggering of anti-gravity muscular patterns, nearly all of the movements he taught to his students were performed lying down.

Despite his background in concrete sciences, Feldenkrais saw beyond what could be scientifically proven. He became interested in the work of Paul Schilder, an Austrian physician and psychiatrist who proposed that habitual reactions involved emotional states, reflexive responses and learned muscular patterns, all of which were intertwined and the triggering of any of which would cause the entire habitual reaction to occur. In other words, he believed that the experience of an emotion includes a physical reaction, and performing a physical action causes the corresponding emotional state to occur.

Feldenkrais witnessed a great deal of anxiety, fear and neuroses in his students. He saw the effects of the withdrawal response, a protective reflex which causes us to contract our flexor muscles when we are frightened or feel defensive. Repeated activation of this reflex, from traumatic events or chronic fear and stress, leads to rounded posture due to habitual contraction of the abdominal muscles. Feldenkrais noticed that his more introverted students tended to have rounded posture, while his extroverted students tended to stand upright.

Feldenkrais observed that when people attempted to correct learned motor habits such as standing with rounded posture, they usually ended up hiding their faulty habits with new habits instead of going through a process of unlearning the faulty habits. He endeavored to create a system which would allow people to directly address and correct dysfunctional movement patterns.

In the mid-twentieth century, the prevailing approach to learning was based on classical conditioning, which had been popularized by Russian physiologist Ivan Pavlov. Classical conditioning begins with a reflex action, and through repetitive training the reflex is triggered simply by the anticipation of a reward. While Pavlov's work with conditioning was significant in showing how environment and external reward can shape behavior, it does not tell the whole story when it comes to man's ability to learn. Classical conditioning gives little to no consideration to the voluntary, conscious processes which occur within our nervous system and how these processes lead to learned behavior.

Feldenkrais realized that the Pavlovian approach to learning as applied to humans was incomplete. Human behavior relies little on reflexes and largely on learned responses, which can become so deeply learned that they feel truly instinctive. He was the first to put together theories of physiology, psychology and neuroscience to create a method by which humans could improve their health and functioning through learning rather than by undergoing physical manipulation or pharmaceutical treatments.

By 1951, Feldenkrais had moved back to Israel to direct the Israeli Army Department of Electronics. Three years later he moved to Tel Aviv and committed himself fully to teaching his techniques of somatic education. He set up a studio where he taught group movement classes in the method he called Awareness Through Movement®. Later in life, he estimated that he had created over a thousand exploratory self-care exercises. The movements combined Gerda Alexander's proprioceptive explorations of sensory awareness with F.M. Alexander's approach of focusing on the process or means-whereby of one's movements. Feldenkrais's refined method was highly effective in improving posture and voluntary motor control. And while he was adamant that he developed his techniques solely for the purpose of sensory-motor education and not to resolve any specific pathologies, his students experienced healing from many functional disorders.

When he moved to Tel Aviv, Feldenkrais began to give private hands-on instruction in addition to his group movement classes. Feldenkrais's hands-on work, which he called Functional Integration®, consisted of two techniques. The first used the principles of means-whereby to give sensory feedback to the student. The student would remain completely passive while Feldenkrais gently moved them through a range of motion, asking them to focus on their internal sensations. This technique allowed the student to become aware of subconscious patterns of muscular tension.

The second technique, which Feldenkrais's student Thomas Hanna later termed "kinetic mirroring," proved to be a major advancement in the field of somatic education. The principle behind kinetic mirroring came from judo, the practice of which was deeply ingrained in Feldenkrais's approach to movement. In judo, one learns not to fight against his opponent's resistance but instead to move with it. Feldenkrais instinctively used this approach when working hands-on with his students. When he felt that a tight muscle was creating resistance, he would move the student's joint or limb in the opposite direction, thereby shortening rather than lengthening the tight muscle. The student remained completely passive while Feldenkrais kept them in this position for a short period of time. After slowly coming out of the position, Feldenkrais found that the tight muscle had begun to relax. It was a wonderful, if somewhat accidental discovery, and the technique became the main method by which Feldenkrais would teach his students how to relax their chronically tight muscles.

It was only later, as Feldenkrais continued his research of neurophysiology, that he came to understand exactly why kinetic mirroring worked. As you learned in Part Two, the resting level of muscular tension is set by the alpha-gamma feedback loop. Let's say that your biceps muscles are contracted about twenty-five percent all the time as a result of weight training. It's impossible for you to completely relax your biceps voluntarily, and you're more comfortable with your elbows bent than straight. When you remain passive and allow someone else to bend your elbow, bringing your biceps into a position that is more than twenty-five percent shortened, that person is effectively doing the work of the muscle; the muscle is being brought into its desired shortened length without having to do any work. Your brain gets the feedback from the Golgi tendon organ that the muscle is shortened and stops sending the message to contract the muscle. This concept can be more easily understood with the example of a thermostat: if a thermostat is set to keep the room at 70 degrees, and the thermostat senses that the temperature has reached 71 degrees, it sends the message to the furnace to shut off. Once the motor neurons have temporarily stopped firing, muscle tension is reduced and the nervous system is more receptive to learning new ways of moving.

In the 1950s and '60s, Feldenkrais traveled around Europe and to the United States to present his work. In 1969, he taught his first teacher training program to twelve students at his studio in Israel. Six years later, he taught his first training in the United States to a group of sixty-five students. Just five years later, in 1980, he began a training in Amherst, Massachusetts which was attended by 235 students. Sadly, he became ill in the fall of 1981 and was unable to complete the program. He passed away in Tel Aviv on July 1, 1984. Feldenkrais left a legacy which is carried on by nearly 3,000 Feldenkrais practitioners all over the world.

Thomas Hanna

Thomas Hanna spent his life in search of freedom. He was born in 1928 in Waco, Texas, so arguably he was free, growing up in one of the freest countries in the world. Yet this eternally curious man sought a different kind of freedom; the kind that comes with internal strength and self-competence, which allows one to be truly autonomous and self-reliant.

Hanna did his undergraduate studies at Texas Christian University, and upon graduating in 1949, decided to pursue his interests in theology and the philosophy of religion—despite being a self-proclaimed atheist. After receiving a Bachelor's degree in Divinity and a doctorate in philosophy from the University of Chicago, Hanna traveled the world teaching, writing, pursuing research, and doing social work. He served as supervisor of an orphanage in Brussels, and directed a club for refugee students at the University of Paris. He was drawn to helping people who, like him, were in search of freedom.

In 1965, Hanna took a position as Chairman of the

Department of Philosophy at the University of Florida. During his travels and his five years in Florida, his continued study of philosophy led him into the fields of psychology, psychotherapy and physiology, which he felt were all deeply connected. While in Florida, Hanna was able to spend a year studying neurology at the University of Florida Medical School. His study of neuroscience taught him that every psychological process occurs along with changes in the systems of the body. It became clear to him that issues of the psyche cannot be fully addressed without working with the functioning of the physical body, and vice versa. He began to refer to the interconnected living process as a "soma," a term which in ancient Greece was used to describe "the living body in its wholeness."

While studying neurology in Florida, Hanna wrote the book *Bodies in Revolt: A Primer in Somatic Thinking*, a survey of somatic philosophy which he published in 1970. After reading this book, an acquaintance told him about the work of Moshe Feldenkrais. Intrigued, Hanna read Feldenkrais's book *Body and Mature Behavior*, and attended his month-long workshop in Berkeley, California in 1973.

During the workshop, Feldenkrais demonstrated his hands-on techniques with a man who had suffered from cerebral palsy since the age of three. The man, then fifty-three, had little control of his movements, and even his voice and breathing were spastic. Feldenkrais asked him to lie down and instructed him to be as passive and relaxed as possible.

Feldenkrais began to instinctively press against the man's

ribcage, gently holding for a short period of time and then changing position. After about twenty minutes of this kinetic mirroring, the man's breathing became slow and smooth, his chest and abdomen rising and falling rhythmically. Feldenkrais then proceeded to work with the man's right hand, which was clenched involuntarily into a fist. Soon the man was able to move his pinky finger independently of his other fingers. Feldenkrais moved up to the man's face and began doing gentle movements with his tongue and jaw. After several minutes, Feldenkrais asked the man to speak, and the words that came out were clear and unstrained. Within just half an hour, Feldenkrais had helped this man begin to unlearn years of habitual muscular patterns which in the eyes of a medical practitioner would have been considered permanent.

Hanna knew in this moment that he wanted to learn how to do what Feldenkrais had just done. At the time, Hanna was the Director of the Humanistic Psychology Institute (now the Saybrook Institute) in San Francisco, and he was able to bring Feldenkrais to the school as a Distinguished Visiting Professor for three years. From 1975 to 1978, Feldenkrais led his professional training program in the United States for the first time, teaching a group of sixty-five students his hands-on method of Functional Integration® and his Awareness Through Movement® exercises.

Feldenkrais's methods gave Hanna the means by which to work with people who suffered from functional disorders and chronic pain conditions. Hanna coined the term "somatic education" to describe methods of education which worked with both the mind and body to improve health and functioning. Inspired to explore the field of somatic education further, Hanna founded the Novato Institute of Somatic Research in Novato, California in 1975.

Hanna observed, just as other somatic educators had, that most adults are quite out of touch with their physical bodies, and likewise that they have lost a great deal of muscular control. Movement is necessary to stimulate the sensory nerves in the muscles and joints, so muscles that do not move are not sensed. It was clear to Hanna that the widespread, nearly pandemic loss of sensation and control was the cause of most functional disorders and chronic pain. He used the term "sensory-motor amnesia" to describe the condition of the central nervous system in which learned, habitual motor patterns have led to chronic muscle contraction and loss of sensation.

Hanna believed that our modern lifestyle is one of the main causes of sensory-motor amnesia. Our survival no longer depends on our physical abilities; the varied movements and active daily lives of our ancestors have been replaced by repetitive tasks and a sedentary way of life. As a result, most people have lost the sensory-motor awareness that comes with frequent, natural and efficient movement. And since this loss of awareness occurs so gradually throughout our lives, most people remain completely unaware that it is occurring until they find themselves in pain or have done actual damage to their bodies. As Hanna wrote in his book *The Body of Life*, "the 'normal' life that most humans lead is a life of unconscious self-destruction."

This self-destruction occurs in different ways and at different rates in each person, but the effects tend to be cumulative and rarely reverse themselves without intervention. Most people appear to be breaking down as they age. We observe this in our loved ones; it makes us fear growing old and even worse, it creates the expectation that we too will begin to fall apart when we reach certain age.

Hanna worked tirelessly to dispel what he called the "myth of aging." This myth tells us that as we age we will cease to be able to do the things we used to do. By ascribing to this myth, we perpetuate it; we stop doing the things we used to, and the result is that we lose the ability to do them. We feel less energetic, our flexibility decreases, our posture and movement become stiff, and we wake up in the morning feeling achy. At some point our structure begins to break down, and we wonder why. The myth of aging is, as Hanna said, "firmly embedded in modern medicine." Our doctors believe it, as medical school offers them no other explanation, and we accept it as fact.

Hanna's study of neurophysiology taught him that the changes we experience in our bodies as we age, instead of being the result of inevitable structural breakdown, are for the most part a result of learning and adaptation. Supported by the latest research which showed that cortical learning occurs throughout our lifetime, Hanna taught his clients that what they had learned could be unlearned. He showed them how to regain sensation and motor control, and they experienced what seemed to be miraculous recoveries from back pain, disc degeneration, sciatica, scoliosis, stooped posture, arthritis, frozen shoulder, and a host of other functional disorders.

Hanna observed that many of his clients' issues were the result of their reactions and adaptations to stress. Feldenkrais had recognized the effects of the withdrawal response, which causes us to adopt a rounded posture when we are frightened or experiencing negative stress. Hanna saw some of his clients exhibit this posture, but observed that other clients tended to arch their back or bend to one side. While Feldenkrais's understanding of how the withdrawal response led to rounded posture was quite accurate, he had no explanation for what caused arched or side-bending postures. Feldenkrais had spent so much of his life focused on defense —to the point that he wouldn't enter a hotel without first finding the escape routes—that he believed that the withdrawal response was the cause of all somatic pathologies.

Hanna had studied the work of endocrinologist Hans Selye, and saw the ways in which Selye's "general adaptation syndrome" related to the functioning of the nervous system. General adaptation syndrome describes a process in which our immediate "fight or flight" response becomes a prolonged, chronic state when we experience long-term stress. When our stress response is activated repeatedly, blood pressure stays elevated, breathing is shallow, levels of certain hormones are increased, cells atrophy, and our neuromuscular responses to stress become learned and automatic to the point that they continue to occur subconsciously even when the stressful stimulus is no longer present.

Selye's work showed that not all stress is caused by negative stimuli. In fact, intense positive emotions and experiences can put the systems of the body under just as much stress as negative ones. Selye coined the term "eustress" to describe positive stress, in contrast to negative stress or "distress."

The concept of eustress explained the contracted back muscles and arched posture that Hanna observed in some of his clients. The muscles in their backs had become chronically tight due to repeated activation of the action response, which is the "fight" part of the fight or flight response. When we experience the kind of stress that makes us want to spring into action, we stand up straight, contracting our back muscles in preparation to move.

Reactions to eustress and distress explained the arched backs and rounded posture that Hanna saw in his clients, but there was a third pattern that did not seem to be the result of stress. Many of Hanna's clients had posture that was tilted to one side or the other, sometimes to the degree that the spinal curvature would be diagnosed as scoliosis. Like the other two postural patterns, Hanna realized that this side bending was the result of an automatic nervous system response which had become learned and habitual. The *flexor reflex*, which makes us contract one side of our body in order to protect it from damage, is triggered constantly when we are recovering from an injury or when we are in pain. When this pattern becomes habitual, the chronic muscular contraction on one side of the body pulls the spine into a C-curve. Sometimes people instinctively balance themselves out by bending to the opposite side, causing them to develop an S-curve in their spine.

During his years at the Novato Institute, Hanna explored movement techniques that would directly address the learned, habitual muscular tension which was the underlying cause of his clients' postural distortions, functional disorders, and chronic pain. He researched the pandicular response, an automatic nervous system response exhibited by vertebrate animals which prevents the buildup of chronic muscle tension. If you've ever seen a dog or cat arch their back when they get up from a nap, or watched a baby stretch their arms and legs as they wake up, you've witnessed the pandicular response. The response involves contracting and releasing muscles in such a way that accurate biofeedback is sent to the brain. This naturally resets the alpha-gamma feedback loop, thereby reducing muscle tension and restoring conscious, voluntary control of the muscles. Essentially, pandiculation "wakes up" the sensory-motor system.

Fetuses have been observed pandiculating while in the womb, showing how deeply ingrained the pandicular response is in our nervous system and how critical it is to our musculoskeletal functioning. Unfortunately, as our motor patterns become habitual and we become less active, our natural pandicular response can't counteract all the learning that is occurring in our nervous system. As we lose sensory-motor awareness and control, our pandicular response can even become inhibited. One of my favorite things that a client has ever said to me is, "You know how my daughter stretches when she wakes up from a nap? I noticed myself doing that this week, and I haven't done that in a very long time!"

Hanna developed hands-on movements and self-care exercises which made use of the pandicular response. He would first teach his clients pandiculations that focused on contracting and releasing one muscle or a small group of muscles, then gradually teach them larger movements which involved moving their entire body. Pandiculation proved to be a groundbreaking movement technique. It quickly reduced muscular tension, and since it relaxed muscles through learning rather than manipulation, the effects were typically long-lasting.

Pandiculation was the first active hands-on technique that a somatic educator had employed to any significant degree. F.M. Alexander had relied on the passive technique of means-whereby, and Feldenkrais used both means-whereby and kinetic mirroring. Through experimentation, Hanna found that voluntary movement on the part of the client was the most efficient and effective way to unlearn chronic, involuntary muscular contraction and form new neural pathways.

Hanna codified his methods into three standard lessons based on the three postural patterns he observed in his clients. He called his approach Clinical Somatic Education. Following each hands-on lesson, Hanna taught his clients simple self-care exercises with the intention that they must learn how to take care of themselves rather than rely on a practitioner to fix them. While Alexander's and Feldenkrais's approaches were free-form, Hanna's was systematized and relatively easy for people to practice at home.

In 1990, after years of people begging him to teach his methods, Hanna began his first professional training program with thirty-eight students. Tragically, after teaching the first semester of the three-semester program, Hanna was killed in a car accident. His students worked with the clients who were on his long waiting list, and went on to create training programs for future students.

Hanna wrote a number of books on somatic education and theory, including the classic *Somatics: Reawakening the Mind's Control of Movement, Flexibility, and Health*. Hundreds of people attended the movement workshops he held in hotel conference centers, and people traveled across the country to do hands-on lessons with him. Hanna created a method of education which not only helped thousands of people get out of pain, but also realized his life's purpose of finding freedom. He freed people from being imprisoned within their stiff, unmoving bodies and gave people the tools with which they could take care of themselves and be truly self-reliant.

* * *

F.M. Alexander, Elsa Gindler, Gerda Alexander and Moshe Feldenkrais were driven to question conventional medical wisdom by a personal need to figure out what was causing their dysfunction. They embarked on highly personal journeys which involved endless hours spent experimenting with how to increase sensation and improve control of their bodies. As science caught up with human experience, it became clear that these pioneers of somatic education had made groundbreaking discoveries about the effect of voluntary control on the functioning of the human nervous system.

In their methods of somatic education we see the process by which each individual solved his or her personal challenge. The Alexander Technique uses subtle shifts in the movement of the head, neck and pelvis to improve posture and function, an approach which enabled F.M. Alexander to regain use of his voice. Elsa Gindler's focus on internal awareness and control of breathing allowed her to recover from tuberculosis, and she taught her students how to improve their health by the same method. Moving with minimal effort and muscular tension enabled Gerda Alexander to regain full function without straining her heart, and these principles became the basis of Eutony.

Feldenkrais approached his problem from a scientific point of view, using his background in engineering and physics to help him figure out why he kept injuring his knees. His combination of scientific knowledge and personal experience led him to create the most effective method of somatic education that had been developed up to that point. However, Feldenkrais's lifelong study of defense gave him a myopic point of view; he believed all dysfunction to be the result of fear and anxiety, and he had difficulty explaining functional issues that were not caused by the withdrawal response.

Hanna benefited from the experiential explorations of all of his predecessors, and since he did not need to satisfy any of his own needs other than curiosity, he was able to approach the work objectively. Developing his techniques thirty years after Feldenkrais and seventy years after F. M. Alexander, Hanna also had access to the latest research in the fields of neuroscience and physiology. As a result, Hanna's method of Clinical Somatic Education proved to be the most comprehensive and effective approach to improving functional disorders.

All of the somatic educators faced the challenge of how to teach their techniques to others. While F.M. Alexander, Gerda Alexander and Feldenkrais established professional training schools, their methods of education were so reliant on personal experience that the lack of an underlying system made it challenging for them to train others. Feldenkrais in particular was a truly gifted practitioner, but had difficulty teaching his hands-on work because he did not fully understand all of the underlying neuromuscular processes that were at work. The experiential, free-form nature of these early methods of somatic education is one of the reasons that the field has not yet become mainstream.

In contrast, Hanna created a highly systematic approach, so teaching his techniques is quite straightforward. Hanna's widow, Eleanor Criswell, and some of his students have dedicated their lives to teaching his work. Yet there are still only an estimated two hundred certified practitioners in the world, so Clinical Somatic Education remains a bit of a secret. When people discover how effective it is, they wonder why they have never heard of it before.

All of the somatic educators firmly believed that their students should not rely on them as any sort of master teacher or guru, but must instead learn to rely on themselves. They wanted people to understand that not only is each individual capable of taking care of their own health, but that it is our responsibility as humans to do so. As Gerda Alexander said in an interview for *Yoga Journal* in 1986:

> *It is better to help people stand on their own two feet, in every sense of the word. It is important, in treatment, not to give and do more than is necessary, so that the other can rely on himself. It is not that I am the great master and give you help. Rather, I can introduce you to my work for your own self discovery.*

Here Alexander describes one of the tenets of somatic education: that the teacher is merely the guide, giving the student the tools with which to increase their sensory-motor awareness, discover the underlying cause of their pain or condition, and improve their physiological functioning.

Another tenet of somatic education is that educators work with students as individual beings rather than on them as indistinguishable physical bodies. A lifetime of different choices, experiences, environments, role models, jobs, injuries and emotional traumas shapes a complex individual who reacts to things in different ways, has unique ideas and thought patterns, and stands and moves like no one else. In Part Two, we talked about the fact that animals are born with most of their motor patterns already in place. Animals' pre-programmed behavior creates a herd of antelope that moves in unison, each animal galloping at the same speed and changing direction simultaneously. While each antelope is nearly indistinguishable from the next, humans are almost infinitely varied in their behavior, movement, posture and physical appearance.

In the following chapters, we will examine the most significant factors that contribute to our development of learned motor patterns: stress, reactions to injuries, repetition of voluntary movements, personality, automatic imitation, and athletic training.

CHAPTER 9

Stress and Posture

If you have any type of chronic or recurring pain, you may have noticed that it tends to become worse with stress. Stress increases overall muscular tension and triggers specific, reflexive postural reactions. And as we learned in Part Two, stress makes us revert to old motor patterns that are deeply learned. So even if you have begun to retrain your patterns, stress can make you slip back into old habits and put you back in pain.

We've already talked about how chronic stress causes changes in brain chemistry, damages brain cells, and leads to conditions such as anxiety and depression, which can worsen the experience of pain. In this chapter we'll discuss the effects of stress on neuromuscular functioning: how the stressors we endure and the ways that we perceive these stressors affect our muscle tension, posture and learned motor patterns.

When we encounter an acute physical stressor, our

automatic fight or flight response is triggered, inducing many physiological changes that prepare us to defend ourselves. The blood vessels that supply our muscles dilate in order to supply extra fuel, and our muscle tension increases so that we can act swiftly and with strength. When the stressor is gone, blood flow slows and our muscle tension returns to normal.

When we experience chronic psychological stress, the same defense mechanisms are triggered. But when our stress response is constantly activated by the ever-present worries in our minds, our neuromuscular system never gets a chance to recover and return to normal. Our heart rate remains elevated and our muscles retain a higher than normal level of tension.

Not surprisingly, studies show that people with anxiety have higher resting levels of muscle tension, react to stress with stronger muscle contractions, and return to their baseline level of tension more slowly than control subjects. As a result of the muscle tension, blood lactate levels are higher in anxiety patients. But what is quite interesting is that it goes both ways: anxiety can be induced by injecting lactate into the bloodstream. So not only does anxiety cause an increased level of muscle tension, but chronic muscular contraction and increased lactate levels can actually cause anxiety.

Just because someone has not been diagnosed with an anxiety disorder does not mean that stress is not a factor in their muscular tension and pain. The level of our psychological stress and the way that we process stress exist on a spectrum. A moderate amount of worry just triggers our stress response to a lesser degree than a diagnosable anxiety condition would. It can be very easy to get used to an increased level of muscle tension and heart rate, and to be completely unaware that your baseline level of stress is elevated.

Even healthy control subjects experience increased and residual tension when they feel stress. One study found that simply having to complete word and math problems in a research lab increased the muscle tension of test subjects. In another experiment, subjects were given a picture and asked to tell a story about it. While they told their stories, their muscle tension increased. When they finished, half of the subjects were praised for doing a good job on the task. Their muscle tension dropped back to normal levels. The other half of the subjects were criticized for their poor performance, and their muscle tension remained higher than normal—until they were reassured by a different researcher that they had actually done a good job.

Mental activity alone, not just psychological stress, is enough to increase muscle tension. Edmund Jacobson, a physician and psychologist, conducted a number of studies in the 1920s and 1930s using an electromyograph (EMG) to observe the correlation between thought and muscle tension. Using a technique he developed called "progressive relaxation" he guided his subjects through a process of contracting and releasing their muscles one by one. As the subjects' muscular tension decreased, their mental activity decreased at the same rate. Once relaxed, it was quite easy to see the elevations in muscle tension that occurred when the subjects were instructed to think about specific things.

When we perceive stress, not only does our overall level

of muscle tension rise, but the withdrawal response and the action response cause us to contract our muscles in predictable patterns depending on whether we perceive the stress to be negative or positive. These responses, like all automatic responses that occur in the human organism, help us survive. The withdrawal response contracts our abdominal muscles to make us curl up in a ball when we are frightened, protecting our internal organs from attack. The action response serves the opposite purpose; it makes us contract our back muscles and stick out our chests, preparing us to move and fight.

While we are born with these automatic responses, experience and learning can affect the degree to which they are activated. If you hear a gunshot, your withdrawal response will automatically be triggered. When you realize that it was just a car backfiring, and you start to hear that same car backfire every day, you'll soon become desensitized to the sound. Your withdrawal response will be activated to a much lesser degree or not at all. This adaptation is generally a good thing—you are adjusting your reaction as a result of learning that the stressor is not dangerous, thus preventing the systems of your body and mind from having to deal with the negative effects of the withdrawal response.

On the flip side, if you perceive a stimulus to be more stressful than it actually is, you may become oversensitized and your automatic responses can increase in frequency and intensity. As you might imagine, this is not a good thing, as it can put a great deal of unnecessary strain on your body and mind.

Moshe Feldenkrais observed the effects of the withdrawal response on posture. His clients who experienced distress on a regular basis and who presented with chronic fear and anxiety were most often the ones who had stooped posture, rounded shoulders, and sunken chests. Thomas Hanna identified the action response as the cause of the opposite posture. His clients who experienced a great deal of eustress, such as those in high-profile jobs who were expected to constantly perform, tended to stand with their backs arched and have chronically contracted back muscles. Hanna concluded that most back and neck pain occurred when people experienced the withdrawal or the action response so frequently that the muscular patterns became habitual.

Distress and Rounded Posture

You're walking down the street and hear gunshots behind you. Within just fourteen milliseconds, your jaw muscles begin to contract. At twenty-five milliseconds, your upper trapezius muscles contract, raising your shoulders and bringing your head forward. At thirty-four milliseconds, the muscles of your eyes and brow contract, squeezing your eyes shut. These lightning-fast neural impulses continue down your body, making your elbows bend, arms rotate inward, abdominal muscles contract, inner thigh muscles and hamstrings tighten, and knees and ankles roll inward. The withdrawal response pulls your extremities inward and brings you into a crouched position, protecting the most vulnerable parts of your body from attack.

Organisms throughout the animal kingdom—amoebas,

earthworms, sea anemones, squirrels, meerkats, sloths, coyotes, monkeys, bears, and of course humans—all exhibit some form of the withdrawal response when danger is sensed. This primitive response occurs automatically and is critical to our survival. In humans and some mammals with more complex nervous systems, the intensity of the response is determined by experience, expectation and baseline stress level.

The withdrawal response has helped us survive and get to where we are today. But for those of us now living in industrialized societies in which our lives are not being threatened on a regular basis, the withdrawal response is not doing us any favors. The never-ending demands of work, family life, financial responsibilities, and social expectations are constantly present in our minds, and we perceive these stressors to be life-threatening. When we experience these types of distress our withdrawal response is activated, contracting our abdominal muscles and bringing us into the rounded posture we associate with aging. When this posture becomes habitual, we experience back and neck pain as well as a host of other physiological dysfunctions including shallow breathing, high blood pressure, and digestive issues. As Moshe Feldenkrais said, "Should the environment change too sharply, the reflex reaction may be the doom of the species as surely as it has served it."

When we experience chronic distress, the muscles involved in the withdrawal response are constantly activated. And we know what happens when we repeat a muscular contraction over and over. Subcortical regions of the brain take control, and over time the pattern of muscular contraction that was originally caused by the withdrawal response becomes habitual; the brain learns to keep those muscles contracted all the time. Now, even if our chronic stress is reduced or eliminated completely, the learned patterns of muscular contraction will remain.

The abdominal muscles are central to the withdrawal response. When they are chronically contracted, the head and ribcage are pulled forward and held there as if we're doing a stomach crunch. Chronic contraction of the abdominals results in *hyperkyphosis*, the rounded posture we associate with aging. Hyperkyphosis occurs when the natural kyphotic curve in the thoracic portion of our spine becomes exaggerated.

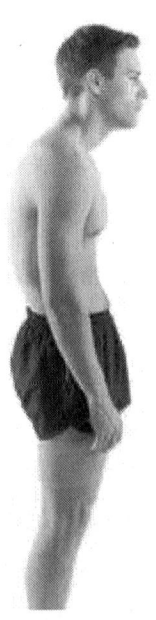

Illustration 4: Hyperkyphosis

This rounded posture is often blamed on osteoporosis, which doesn't make a whole lot of sense. Bones don't move out of alignment unless muscles tell them to, and the fact that bones have become weak and brittle does not directly affect whether we adopt a rounded, straight or arched posture.

People with what is often referred to as "forward head posture" are shown to have significantly more neck pain and disability than people with normal posture, and the further forward they hold their head, the greater their pain. For every inch your head moves forward, it effectively gains ten pounds in weight because of the increased strain on the muscles of your neck and upper back. Your suboccipital muscles, just below the base of your skull, must contract even further if you want to lift your head up to face forward instead of looking down at the ground. Pain can result simply from all of these muscles being chronically contracted, and in addition, disc problems and nerve pain may develop from the increased compression of the cervical spine.

Hyperkyphosis can also cause back pain. When your abdominals contract and the weight of your head and ribcage are pulled in front of your center of gravity, you quite literally will fall forward if you don't do something to balance yourself out. So as your abdominals gradually become habitually contracted, your back muscles must work harder and harder to keep you upright in gravity. A person with hyperkyphosis may complain only of a sore back, but all attempts to treat the back muscles directly will have little effect until the underlying cause—the habitual abdominal contraction—is addressed.

In addition to causing pain and disc degeneration, chronically contracted abdominals have negative effects on many other functions of the body. Tight abdominals limit the ability to take a full breath, which demands that the diaphragm be able to contract downward and push the contents of the abdomen forward. If the abdominals are tight, this action cannot occur and breathing becomes shallow and strained. Chronic tightness and compression in the front of the body also puts pressure on all the internal organs, contributing to high blood pressure, digestive problems, frequent urination, constipation and impotence.

The abdominal muscles are the strongest and most central muscles acting in the withdrawal response. However, habitual contraction of the internal rotators and flexor muscles of the extremities can cause health problems as well. The withdrawal response contracts the inner thigh muscles, rotating the thighs inward; this places stress on the knees and ankles and makes the arches of the feet collapse. Hip flexors, quadriceps and hamstring muscles become tight and sore from holding the body in a flexed position. Headaches, teeth grinding, TMJ disorders, and bruxism (ringing in the ears) can develop due to constant contraction of the neck and jaw muscles.

The effects of the withdrawal response tend to be more obvious in the elderly, simply because they have been alive longer and have had more exposure to stress. But there are two important things to note here. One, it is not inevitable that we will develop rounded posture as we age. The way that we perceive and cope with stress throughout our lives determines how the systems of our body react. Learning how to deal with stress in a constructive way can prevent you from automatically triggering your withdrawal response and suffering the negative physical effects.

Two, we can develop rounded posture at any age. There is a fairly recent shift in our daily lives that has caused many people to begin developing hyperkyphosis during their twenties and thirties, teens and even earlier. I am talking about the advent of personal computers, smart phones, and the myriad of other devices which keep us constantly connected and entertained. Spending hours upon hours sitting at a computer keeps us in the withdrawal response posture: hips and knees flexed, arms rotated inward, and head forward. It takes a great deal of conscious attention, as well as proper seating, to prevent this posture from becoming habitual.

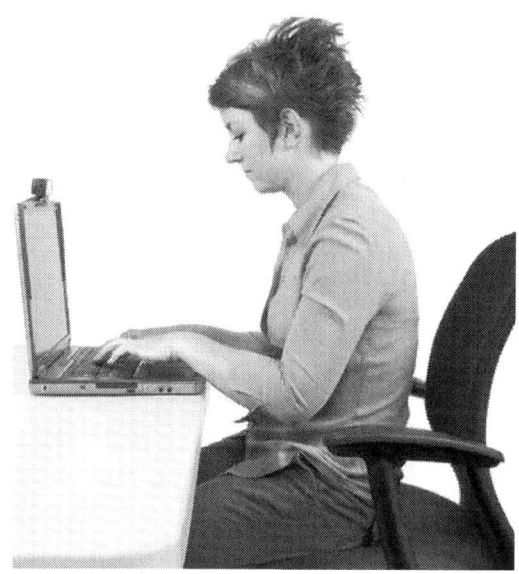

Illustration 5: Typical Computer Posture

We only need to walk around a shopping mall to observe the effects of smart phones and a sedentary lifestyle on young people. It is fairly impossible to use a smart phone without looking downward and contracting the biceps and pectoral muscles, and when you consider that the average person between the ages of eleven and eighteen spends eight hours and twenty minutes per day using some form of electronic media, it is easy to see how quickly rounded posture can become habitual. It always makes me sad to see a lovely teenager in the prime of their life who has already begun to round forward as if they are eighty years old.

In addition to new technology and changes in daily activities, our competitive, industrialized society puts ever-increasing demands on children and teenagers. We subject them to the same social constructs and pressure to succeed that we face as adults. As a result, their stress responses—most often their withdrawal response—are triggered far more often than in past generations.

There are still other factors which contribute to rounded posture. Fatigue, which in and of itself is often stressful, makes us want to curl up in a ball and go to sleep. Chronic lack of sleep alone can cause someone to slouch and adopt the withdrawal response posture. People who are quite tall often develop rounded posture as a result of functional needs like working at a counter top built for average height people, or as a result of feeling insecure and wanting to fit in by shortening their stature. Abdominal surgery or injury often results in withdrawal response posture, as people instinctively want to protect the painful area by contracting the muscles around it.

Athletic training that demands a great deal of core strength, such as swimming or gymnastics, can cause even the most highly trained athletes to have rounded shoulders and sunken chests. And simply being cold on a regular basis can contribute to withdrawal response posture. Notice what happens next time you feel really cold: you'll bring your arms in toward your body, round your shoulders and raise them up, and if you're sitting or lying down you'll contract your abdominals and curl up into the fetal position to stay warm.

Eustress and the Arched Back

In the first few months of life the human infant is entirely helpless, unable to crawl or even sit up by himself. He has spent nine months curled up in the fetal position and has yet to gain control of the extensor muscles of his neck and back. Around three months of age, he will finally succeed in lifting his head off the ground when lying on his stomach. A few months later, the muscles in his lower back are activated, allowing him to crawl, sit up, and eventually stand and walk.

Once he is using the extensor muscles of his back and neck on a regular basis, the cervical and lumbar curves in his spine will begin to develop. These are called lordotic curves, and they curve in the opposite direction as the kyphotic curves of the thoracic and sacral portions of the spine. The natural kyphotic and lordotic curves of the spine are essential to the spine's ability to absorb shock; they allow the spine to function like a big spring. If we didn't have these curves, our vertebrae would be stacked on top of each other in a straight line, and compressive forces would cause a great deal of damage and pain.

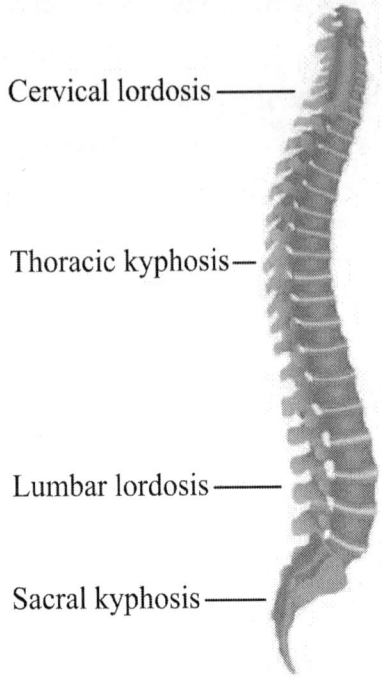

Illustration 6: Natural Spinal Curvature

In infants, the contraction of the back and neck muscles in response to the instinctive desire to become mobile is called the Landau Reflex. But even after we learn how to stand, walk and run, our extensor muscles automatically contract every time we want to get up and go; this is the action response. We arch our back, lift our head, pull our shoulders backward, stick out our chests, straighten our knees, and rotate our legs outward.

Our action response is also triggered by eustress, or positive stress, such as giving a presentation or meeting our new boss. Whenever we want to make a good impression and be on our game, we instinctively contract our back muscles so that we stand up straight, look taller, and appear to be confident. This posture prepares us both physically and psychologically for action.

We subconsciously associate this upright, often arched posture with confidence, strength, youth and beauty. It is no coincidence that the military trains soldiers to stand up straight and stick out their chests. The action response posture shows the enemy that they are ready for a fight. And we find it much more pleasing to look at someone who stands erect rather than rounded over; imagine watching a dancer or ice skater who was slouching as they performed.

So far, the action response sounds pretty great. It prepares us for action and automatically makes us look and feel more confident—and all in a completely natural way. But you probably know where I'm going with this. When our action response is triggered once in a while, it is great. But when it's activated constantly by a high-stress job or practiced repetitively as part of physical training, the pattern of muscular contraction becomes learned. So even after you retire from your stressful job or quit dancing, your back muscles remain habitually tight, causing soreness, pain, and often structural damage to intervertebral discs.

When the extensor muscles of the back are chronically contracted, they will typically pull the lumbar spine into hyperlordosis. The exaggerated arching of the lower back compresses the discs in between the lumbar vertebrae, often causing the discs to bulge or herniate. People with tight lower back muscles may experience sciatica due to compression of the sciatic nerve as it exits the spine in between the lumbar vertebrae. Tight lower back muscles also compress the sacroiliac joint, causing pain and inflammation, and occasionally shifting the joint out of alignment.

Once the action or withdrawal response has become habitual, and we are subconsciously holding ourselves in a dysfunctional posture most or all of the time, pain becomes pretty much inevitable. Research shows that people who stand with an arched back, flat back, or sway back are all more likely to experience pain than people who stand with normal posture. Luckily, as somatic educators have discovered, this pain can be alleviated and eliminated by unlearning the damaging postural patterns.

Aging and The Dark Vise

We all experience both the action response and the withdrawal response throughout our lifetimes, in varying frequencies and to different degrees, depending on the stressors we encounter and the ways that we perceive them. In the moment of a strong reaction to an acute stressor, the reflex pattern of muscular contraction can be fairly pure, bringing our body into a full expression of the action response or withdrawal response posture. Each time the posture is repeated, just a small degree of it is retained in our muscle memory. Over time, our individual responses to stress contribute to patterns of posture and movement that are completely, uniquely ours.

The muscular contractions of the action response and the withdrawal response work against each other. The action response cues the nervous system to automatically release the flexors of the body so as to allow for unhindered contraction of the extensors. The withdrawal response has the opposite effect, automatically releasing the extensors so that the flexors can curl the body up into the fetal position.

As we age, we tend to become increasingly immobile as these opposing muscular patterns fight against each other. Both the abdominal muscles and the lower back muscles pull the ribcage down toward the pelvis, compressing our spine and shortening our stature. Our trunk, which once bent and twisted freely, becomes stiff and unmoving. Our natural ability to balance ourselves with contralateral movement is now limited. One only needs to watch a young person walk next to their grandparent in order to observe the effects of muscular rigidity that occur with age. Notice how the young person moves with ease, their trunk twisting and limbs swinging freely, while their grandparent moves quite stiffly.

Thomas Hanna called this gradual locking down of the body the "dark vise." So slowly that it is barely noticeable, we tighten up like a vice grip, pulling ourselves inward and downward toward our center. Our muscles and connective tissues tighten, our movement becomes constricted, and waking up feeling stiff and achy is the norm.

To add insult to injury, all of this chronic muscular contraction has another adverse effect: chronic fatigue. As we learned in Part One, muscles require energy in order to contract. The more muscle tension we have, the more energy we are continually expending, and the more tired we become. Even a full night's sleep does not feel refreshing because our muscles have stayed partially contracted throughout the night, using up energy while we sleep.

* * *

We can't avoid the withdrawal response or the action response completely, nor would we want to—they still come in handy sometimes. But we do need to become acutely aware of when these responses are being triggered and the impact they are having on our posture, movement and pain. Because while getting locked down into the dark vise is not inevitable, the reality is that it is quite likely to happen to some degree unless we are very self-aware and take conscious action to prevent it.

Research consistently shows the correlation between stress and pain. But even more important than the type or amount of stressors we encounter is the way that we individually deal with stress. We each perceive and cope with stress differently due to our personality and past experiences. A stressful occurrence that might trigger the action response in one person could trigger the withdrawal response in someone else, and another person might not perceive the occurrence to be stressful at all. Becoming aware of your reactions to stress and learning how to modify them is one of the most important things you can do to prevent pain caused by muscular tension and postural responses.

CHAPTER 10

Injury, Handedness and Scoliosis

Imagine that you've slipped on your icy front steps and sprained your ankle. On top of the fact that you don't have an exciting mountaineering story to tell, you have to wear an ankle brace and use crutches for at least a month so that the torn ligaments can heal. You have to put all your weight on your uninjured side, and you instinctively contract and immobilize the injured side in order to protect it. Over the next four weeks, you get really good at hobbling around on your one good leg. This unnatural way of moving starts to become habitual, and even after your ankle is fully healed, you find yourself standing with your weight shifted to one side and the other hip hiked up.

Now imagine that you have chronic pain in your right shoulder. The doctors say you have a torn rotator cuff, a result of years of wear and tear from weight lifting. As the pain increases, you use your shoulder less and less in order to avoid the pain, and develop the tendency to hold your right arm against your body to limit the movement in your shoulder. After surgery and months of physical therapy, your pain is finally gone, but your learned movement pattern remains. The muscles that hold your shoulder in place and pull your arm in toward your body are chronically contracted, and your right shoulder is now an inch lower than your left.

The ways that we adjust our posture and movement in reaction to an injury or chronic pain are largely subconscious. We contract certain muscles to protect the painful or injured area, and modify our motor patterns to avoid the pain. Our pain processing system works with our proprioceptive and vestibular systems to automatically adjust our posture and movement so that we can minimize our pain and prevent further injury.

When one side of the body is injured or feels pain, such as when you step on a nail or touch a very hot pan, an automatic nervous system response called the *flexor reflex* is triggered. The flexor muscles on the injured side of your body contract to pull the affected area away from the source of pain. Then the *crossed-extensor reflex* immediately kicks in, activating the extensor muscles on the opposite side of your body so that your weight remains balanced and you don't fall over.

The flexor reflex is extremely helpful during acute pain or injury because it helps us avoid pain and further damage to our body. However, when it is activated constantly by chronic pain or a prolonged healing process from an injury, we can easily develop motor patterns that stay with us permanently.

What begins as a protective postural mechanism becomes a habitual motor pattern, causing misalignment, dysfunctional movement, and further pain. Our heightened emotional state during and after an injury also contributes to the pattern getting locked in. Much like never forgetting our marriage proposal even though it only occurs once, a strong emotional reaction can cause a pattern to become deeply learned immediately.

Our reflexive, protective response to injury will always be experienced on one side unless our injury or pain is directly in the center of our body, such as in our abdomen or along our spine. For example, after abdominal surgery we will tend to stand with rounded posture in order to protect our abdomen, which has effectively gone through trauma. Likewise, if our spine is injured our back muscles will tighten up in order to limit movement.

Thomas Hanna observed the effects of the flexor reflex in his clients: tilted and often rotated posture, uneven hips and shoulders, and different patterns of muscular contraction on each side of the body. Many of these clients had sciatica or pain in their hip, knee and ankle joints, while others had frozen shoulder, bursitis or carpal tunnel syndrome. Some of them had even been told by doctors that they had one leg longer than the other. This perceived difference in leg length was caused by tight waist muscles hiking one hip up higher than the other. When Hanna taught his clients how to release their oblique muscles, their hips evened out and miraculously, their legs were the same length.

Handedness

In addition to injury, an important factor in determining how we use the two sides of our bodies is our handedness. Whether we are right- or left-handed plays a large role in the movement patterns we develop. It determines how we sit at our desk and use our computer, which shoulder we carry our bag on, which leg we kick a ball with, and which side we tend to lean on.

We refer to our sides as being dominant and non-dominant, but in reality, both sides of our body play equally important roles in our ability to carry out complicated motor tasks. If we are right-handed, we tend to use our right side to perform tasks requiring precision and dexterity, while our left side plays the critical role of providing support and balance. We develop patterns of habitual muscular contraction on both sides of our bodies. On our dominant side, the tension is the result of repetition of voluntary movement, and on our non-dominant side, it is the result of automatically holding and stabilizing.

It is not only useful, but necessary and entirely human to use the sides of our bodies in different ways. Unfortunately, when our motor patterns become strengthened by a great deal of repetition or lifting of heavy weights, or when our reaction to an injury enhances our patterns, we can find ourselves out of balance to the point that we are in pain and causing damage to the structure of our body. It is very important to notice when we are overdoing one-sided movements, and to teach ourselves to use the sides of our body more evenly. We'll talk about how to do this in Part Four.

Scoliosis

Both our natural reaction to physical trauma and our handedness can contribute to the condition of scoliosis, which is a lateral (side-bending) of the spine. Scoliosis most often occurs when tight muscles pull the spine out of alignment. Recall that there are natural lordotic and kyphotic curves in the spine which help to absorb shock, and when these curves increase to an atypical degree, they are called hyperlordosis and hyperkyphosis. Scoliosis is different; there is no natural lateral curve in the spine, so any degree of side-bending can be considered dysfunctional.

Scoliosis is regarded as a mysterious, incurable condition by most of the medical community. While some cases are clearly present at birth or caused by diseases such as cerebral palsy or muscular dystrophy, the vast majority—between eighty and eighty-five percent—are classified as idiopathic. In other words, the cause of most scoliosis cases is unknown.

Between two and four percent of teenagers are diagnosed with scoliosis, while more than eight percent of adults over the age of forty are diagnosed. The fact that scoliosis becomes more prevalent with age is a strong indicator that our learned motor patterns, the effects of which increase over time, play a role in developing the condition. And interestingly, ninety percent of adolescent thoracic scoliosis cases curve to the right, and around ninety percent of the population is right-handed. This suggests that the way people habitually use the sides of their bodies due to their handedness can determine the direction of their scoliotic curves.

While some cases of scoliosis are caused by structural

deformity, the majority are caused by muscles pulling the spine out of alignment. Chronic muscular contraction on one side of the spine pulls the vertebrae into a C-shaped curve, and contraction on both sides causes an S-curve. Typically, a curve of eleven degrees or more will garner a diagnosis of scoliosis. If the curve is greater than twenty to twenty-five degrees, a brace will be prescribed. If the curve progresses to more than forty-five degrees, spinal fusion surgery will most likely be recommended.

Roughly two-thirds of adults with scoliotic curves between twenty and fifty-five degrees experience back pain. Many people with scoliosis develop pain in other parts of their bodies as well due to their postural misalignment, which puts uneven stress on the hips, knees, neck and shoulders. Arthritis, disc and nerve compression in the spine, and difficulty breathing are also common.

About 38,000 scoliosis patients in the United States undergo spinal fusion surgery each year. In spinal fusion surgery, metal rods, hooks, wires and screws are attached to the spine in order to force it into a straight position. Then doctors attach pieces of bone, which grow together and create the actual fusion of the spine. Patients who undergo this type of surgery lose twenty to sixty percent of their spinal flexibility. A great deal of strain is put on the unfused parts of the spine, leading to a high rate of disc degeneration and osteoarthritis. Research shows that seventy-five percent of patients experience degeneration in their sacroiliac joint after spinal fusion surgery. And sadly, more than forty percent of spinal fusion patients experience no reduction in their pain levels.

Rates of complications in spinal fusion surgeries vary, but are quite high across the board. Some research has shown that more than half of the surgeries are unsuccessful, meaning that the vertebrae do not actually fuse. Even though the vertebrae are held in place by hardware, patterns of contraction in the back muscles cause micromovements in the spine, preventing continuous growth of the bone. Muscular contraction can be so strong that the metal rods that are inserted along the spine can actually break, causing a great deal of pain and requiring repeat surgery. Given the high risk of complications and the lack of evidence supporting spinal fusion as an effective treatment, many doctors and researchers now agree that the surgery can be used to slow or halt progression of the curvature, but little else.

In fact, attempting to improve a functional issue like a spinal curve by using manual force is fairly ludicrous. When a bone is broken, it is a structural issue, and the bone must be manually set in place in order to heal. But when the skeleton is pulled out of alignment by the muscles, it is a functional issue; the way that the nervous system is functioning is causing the misalignment. Using a brace or metal rods to force the spine into alignment will have little to no effect on the messages that the nervous system is sending to the muscles to contract. Scoliosis patients who learn how to release the chronic muscular contraction that is causing their curvature typically experience reduction or elimination of pain as well as gradual straightening of their spine.

* * *

Now that you have learned about the effects of the withdrawal response, action response and flexor reflex, you will likely find it difficult not to notice them in everyone you see. You'll observe strangers on the street hunched over, their backs and shoulders rounded and their heads sticking forward. You'll be able to tell who among your friends has back pain simply by observing their tight, arched lower backs. You may even look in the mirror and see that one of your shoulders or hips is higher than the other. Don't worry—these are all functional issues that can be improved and eliminated with the methods of Clinical Somatic Education that I'll discuss in Part Four.

CHAPTER 11

The Daily Grind

We've already talked about how repetition of a voluntary, conscious movement pattern leads to that pattern becoming automatic and subconscious. There are countless examples of repetitive activities that we do in our daily lives—brushing our teeth, talking on the phone, carrying a baby, working on an assembly line, and lifting heavy objects—that lead us to develop habitual ways of using our bodies. Let's examine a situation that I believe most people can relate to: carrying a bag on one shoulder.

You likely started carrying a bag to school on a daily basis when you entered kindergarten. There's a pretty good chance that you carried a backpack on both shoulders. But at some point, whether out of convenience or trying to look cool, this habit probably shifted into carrying the backpack, duffel, tote bag or purse on just one side.

When you first started carrying the bag on one shoulder,

you likely chose which side to carry it on based on whether you are right or left-handed. The more often you carried your bag on that same shoulder, the more comfortable it became. And without knowing it, you instinctively adjusted your entire posture in order to keep that bag on your shoulder. If you were carrying the bag on your right side, you pulled your right shoulder backward and held your right arm still to prevent the bag from slipping off your shoulder. This resulted in a subtle twisting of your entire torso to the right. You also shifted your ribcage to the left and put more weight on your left leg to balance out the weight of the bag.

Believe it or not, you make these postural adjustments every time you carry a bag on one side, even if it is small and lightweight. You make similar adjustments every time you carry anything on one side. Try standing up and holding a bag on one shoulder as you typically do. Then try holding it on the other shoulder. You might feel uncoordinated, and it might even feel as though it is impossible to hold it on this side.

When I ask my clients to try carrying their bag on their other shoulder, they usually look at me and say, "But...I can't." The postural adjustments involved in carrying a bag on one shoulder are so deeply learned that it truly feels as though they are physically unable to do the opposite.

You might be asking yourself—why is this such a big deal? To a certain extent, it's not. Virtually all of us are right- or left-handed, and as a result we develop movement patterns in which we use the two sides of our bodies differently. This is a natural part of the way that humans move, and it allows us to perform complex tasks.

However, like any motor pattern, this habit becomes problematic when it is repeated too often or under the strain of too much weight. Carrying a bag on the same shoulder every day of your life can cause the postural adjustments involved to become so deeply learned that you stand and move that way all the time: one shoulder pulled up and back, spine twisted to one side, and ribcage and weight shifted to the other side.

As you already know, when an unnatural pattern becomes habitual, you tend to become increasingly unaware of it. This lack of awareness allows you to fall deeper and deeper into that pattern until at some point, the pattern becomes dysfunctional enough that it begins to cause problems. You could feel run-of-the-mill muscle pain, but you could also feel something more serious such as a pinched nerve or joint pain due to cartilage being worn away. Pain and damage to the structure of your body—all due to a learned movement pattern which has likely been developing since childhood.

In the past, chronic pain and postural changes were typically seen in adults middle-aged and older, and as a result these issues were assumed to be an inevitable part of the aging process. But over the past fifty years or so, with the advent of television, video games, personal computers and smart phones, we have begun to see back pain, neck pain, and dysfunctional postural habits commonly occurring in teens and even children.

A study of over eight hundred Australian teenagers found that computer use was associated with habitual postural deviations such as increased head and neck flexion (meaning that their heads tilted forward and down). The flexion was consistent whether the teens were looking straight ahead, looking downward, sitting in a slumped position, or standing up. At their young age, the teenagers' postural habits were already so deeply learned that their heads and necks remained flexed even when they weren't at the computer.

The study also found associations between small variations in posture and increased neck and shoulder pain. Slight changes in habitual posture can be enough to cause pain, even in young people who are typically quite resilient and feel little pain. This is why carrying your bag on the same shoulder every day is such a big deal; you never know what seemingly meaningless movement habit might be causing or contributing to your pain.

Stop and think for a few minutes about motor patterns you have developed over the years as a result of the repetition of voluntary movements and postures. Think about the way you sit or move at work, the way you drive, the way you talk on the phone, and how you sit to read or watch television. Also think about any movement pattern that you have put conscious energy into learning, whether it be for athletics, playing an instrument, or completing a task at work. Do you think that any of your movement habits might be contributing to your pain?

CHAPTER 12

Personality

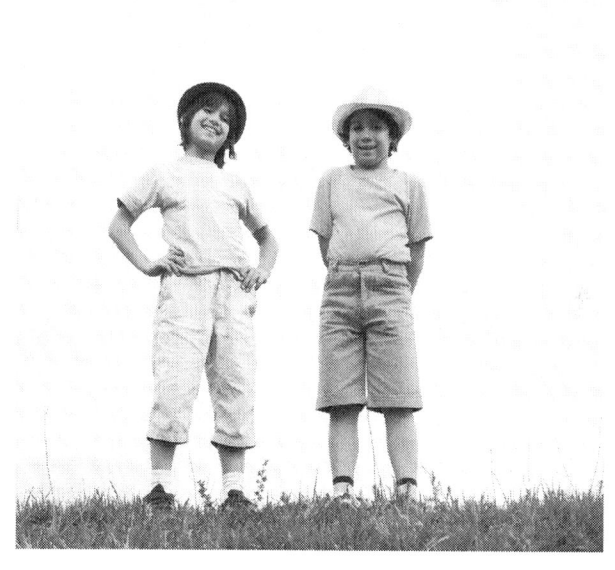

Illustration 7: Personality and Posture

Take a look at this photo of two young boys. The boy on the left is relaxed and quite confident, happy to be the center of attention and to have his picture taken. We can literally see how he is feeling by observing his body language. He stands with his pelvis pushed forward and his hands on his hips, opening up his chest and abdominal area. His relaxed stance and easy smile show that he has no worries and is not feeling defensive.

In contrast, the boy on the right is shy and nervous. He's forcing a smile, clearly trying to put on a brave face even though he wishes he could get away from the camera. The boy's upper back is rounded, his chest concave and his shoulders raised, all of which are reflexive postural reactions to feeling afraid. If confronted by a bully, this boy would likely run the other way—unless his buddy on the left stepped in to defend him first.

How can we tell all this from a photo? Because our postures, facial expressions and movements communicate the way we feel inside. Scientists have found that somewhere between sixty and ninety-three percent of all communication is non-verbal. This helps explain our desire to use multiple exclamation points and emoticons when sending emails and text messages. When we can't communicate face-to-face, written words are not enough—we need to rely on symbols to convey our emotions. And interestingly, our subconscious use of body language isn't limited to direct communication with others. Our emotional state is constantly being conveyed through our posture and the way we move, even if we are alone and no one can see us.

If we want to trick someone or make a good impression, we often instinctively try to fake our body language, like the boy in the picture who is smiling despite feeling uncomfortable. In the boy's case, however, his smile is not convincing enough to hide his habitual posture. His withdrawal reflex has been triggered so many times that he is now stuck in that posture involuntarily all the time.

Like any habitual motor pattern, we can change our body language through intentional practice and repetition. And by changing our body language, we can actually change the way we feel inside. Amy Cuddy of Harvard University and Dana Carney and Andy Yap of Columbia University tested the effects of what they call "power posing," and the results of their research have fascinating, real-world applications. In the study, test subjects had to spend two minutes sitting in high-power poses or low-power poses. High-power poses were expansive and open, meaning that the subject expanded their body to take up more space and brought their limbs away from the center of their body. Subjects in low-power poses took up less space and brought their limbs in closer to the center of their body. These postures should sound familiar: the action response triggers high-power poses, and the withdrawal response brings us into low-power poses.

The study measured levels of cortisol and testosterone before and after power posing. Levels of the stress hormone cortisol is typically higher in people who people who feel powerless, and lower in those who feel powerful. The steroid hormone testosterone is linked to assertiveness, and people with high levels of testosterone typically feel powerful and act confidently.

The effects of spending just two minutes in either high-power or low-power poses yielded significant results. The high-power posers experienced a spike in testosterone levels and a drop in cortisol levels, while the low-power posers experienced a drop in testosterone and a rise in cortisol. These hormone changes were accompanied by emotional shifts; the high-power posers reported feeling more powerful and were more likely to take a gambling risk after striking their poses than the low-power posers. Incredibly, spending just two minutes in a posture has immediate effects on the way we feel, our behavior, and even our hormone levels. Imagine the effects of spending a lifetime in a certain posture.

Power posing even affects how we perceive pain. Researchers from the University of Toronto and the University of Southern California explored how adopting a dominant or submissive pose might affect a person's pain tolerance. Their results were quite clear: test subjects had an increased tolerance for pain after holding a dominant pose for just twenty seconds. One reason for this is the sense of control that power posing elicits. Studies have shown that when we perceive that we have control over a situation, our tolerance for pain increases. Likewise, when we feel that we're not in control, we have a reduced tolerance for pain. A second reason that power posing affects pain tolerance is its effect on levels of testosterone; higher levels of testosterone increase our tolerance for pain.

What we are building up to is that our personality—the unique combination of emotional and behavioral characteristics that make us who we are—causes us to adopt certain postures and movement patterns. We repeat these patterns over and over, and gradually they become deeply learned habits. Over time, the learned patterns themselves contribute to the way we feel and behave. Our personality and our learned motor patterns work in tandem to keep us stuck in habitual ways of standing, moving, feeling and acting.

Can we then predict what habitual postural patterns a person will develop based on their personality? It appears that to some degree, the answer is yes. In a study comparing personality and posture, researchers from McGill University and the San Diego University for Integrative Studies found striking correlations between posture and extraverted versus introverted personality traits.

The researchers separated their test subjects into groups based on four different habitual postures: ideal posture, kyphosis-lordosis posture (in which the kyphotic and lordotic curves of the spine are exaggerated), sway back (in which the lumbar curve of the spine is decreased and the hips are in front of the ankles), and flat back (in which the lumbar portion of the spine is flat). The study showed that ninety-six percent of the subjects who had ideal posture and eighty-three percent of the subjects who had kyphosis-lordosis posture were extraverts. The introverts, on the other hand, were far more likely to stand with either a sway back or flat back. These results are quite remarkable, especially when you look at the position of the lower back and pelvis in these postures. The extraverts tended to hold their pelvis upright or tipped forward, resulting in a natural or enhanced arch in their lower back. In other words, the people who were more confident and outgoing had adopted the powerful posture of the action response. In contrast, the introverts had a strong tendency to contract their abdominal muscles and tuck their pelvis under —the submissive posture of the withdrawal response— creating a flattening of the natural lumbar curve and bringing them into flat back or sway back posture.

The study also found that the muscles of people who had ideal posture were more relaxed, and the muscles of those who had the three non-ideal postures were more contracted. This should come as no surprise because as you have already learned, our muscles have to actively work to keep us in an unnatural posture. Predictably, the people who had the three non-ideal postures also experienced more back and neck pain than those who had ideal posture.

So, our personalities play a role in the motor patterns that we develop. And our motor patterns affect the way we feel inside and how we behave, especially once the patterns have become habitual and we are standing and moving in these patterns all the time. And unfortunately, these patterns lead to increased muscle tension and sometimes pain and actual physical damage to our body.

Consider how your thoughts and emotions may have contributed to your habitual posture and movement. Also, start noticing when certain motor patterns are triggered and how they affect you. For example, do you notice that when you feel powerless you slouch, letting your chest collapse and shoulders round? Does this put strain on your neck, shoulders or lower back? Noticing patterns like this will help you to become more aware of how your personality and body language are working together, and how they may be putting you in pain.

CHAPTER 13

Automatic Imitation

You're interviewing for a new job and the competition is stiff. Your potential new boss, Mr. Peterson, leans forward in his chair, gesturing passionately as he discusses the issues his company is facing. You lean forward, listening intently and responding with equally strong ideas and gestures. Mr. Peterson then leans back in his chair and asks you to explain your thoughts further. You lean back and go into detail about your plan to get the company back on track.

Liking what he's hearing, Mr. Peterson crosses his legs and leans on his right elbow. You settle into the same posture and continue to explain your plan. The two of you discuss the future of the company, each nodding along as the other talks. As you leave, Mr. Peterson thinks to himself, "I really liked that guy. He had great ideas and I felt like we were on the same page."

You've successfully nailed the interview, thanks in large

part to your instinctive use of automatic imitation. Your strong desire to establish rapport with Mr. Peterson made you subconsciously mimic his body language. As a result, he felt a connection with you, was receptive to your ideas, and genuinely liked you.

While psychologists have been observing and discussing automatic imitation in many species since the mid-eighteenth century, it wasn't until recently that the underlying mechanism of the behavior became clear. In the 1990s, Italian neuroscientist Giacomo Rizzolatti and a group of researchers at the University of Parma discovered a type of brain cells in monkeys known as mirror neurons. Then in 2010, researchers at UCLA made the first recording of single mirror neurons in the human brain.

Mirror neurons, which are found in parts of the brain responsible for movement, vision and memory, are activated equally when we perform an action and when we observe another person performing an action. Like pretty much everything that happens automatically in our nervous system, the way these neurons function help us to survive. Automatically imitating other people's postures and movements helps to establish a sense of affinity and facilitate communication, both of which are vital elements in forming relationships and creating a healthy group dynamic.

Automatic imitation also plays a role in our ability to perceive others' emotions, an essential skill in maintaining relationships and communicating. We know this thanks to Botox, a highly toxic substance which keeps muscles relaxed by blocking signals from motor nerves to the muscles. When test subjects are given facial injections of Botox, both their ability to mimic facial expressions and their ability to perceive emotions are impaired. Sensory feedback from muscular contraction in facial expressions is critical to our ability to understand what others are feeling.

We tend to subconsciously imitate the people with whom we spend a great deal of time and have a desire to create rapport. As we initially develop motor patterns during childhood, we subconsciously imitate our family members' posture and movement. So if you think you get your posture from your mother, you could be right—but genetics doesn't have much to do with it. Automatic imitation is so dependent on social relationships that animals even imitate their human owners. Recent studies have shown that dogs yawn contagiously when their owners yawn, and that they can't help imitating their owners' actions even when a food reward should compel them to do the opposite.

Groups of teenagers often display a great deal of automatic imitation due to their strong desire to fit in and be accepted. Teenagers want so badly to be part of a group that their subconscious minds work overtime to create similarities between themselves and their peers. At this age, habitual postures learned from friends may tend to override those learned from parents and siblings.

As adults, new motor patterns are formed as we subconsciously imitate our spouse. Mirror neurons fire when we merely observe someone we want to connect with, so simply spending time with your spouse can lead to changes in your posture and movement. As you walk down the street, notice couples who walk at the same pace, with the same gait and same posture.

Take a few moments to think about how your motor patterns may have been shaped by close family members, friends and your spouse. And as you go through your daily life, notice how you automatically mirror other people's body language while talking to or spending time with them. You may be surprised by the degree to which automatic imitation affects the way you stand and move.

CHAPTER 14

Training Pain

You and the pitcher are staring each other down, motionless, each trying to read the others mind. You watch him shift his weight, wind up and release the ball. A moment later, you hear the crack of your bat hitting the ball, and watch the ball soar off into center field. Your brain took in everything you saw about the pitcher's preparation, made the decision about what type of swing would be most likely to hit his pitch, and sent messages to your muscles to contract in a specific, complex sequence—all in less than half a second.

During a game, competition or performance, there is little time for conscious decision-making; every reaction must happen both instantaneously and accurately. This is why athletes practice so much. It's not just about being in the best possible physical condition. It's about training the entire neuromuscular system to be able to react automatically and with precision while under stress.

Athletes spend so much time consciously training themselves with the goal of acquiring muscle memory that their motor patterns tend to be very deeply learned. And depending on what sport or discipline they practice, they may have to train themselves to move in unnatural ways. Athletes' movement patterns are also shaped by stress, personality, and all of the other factors we've already talked about. When combined with the training required by their chosen sport, the result is that their patterns can more complex than non-athletes.

Sometimes athletic training will improve an individual's posture and movement, helping to correct imbalances and increase overall strength and flexibility. But in many cases, the great number of repetitions or the strain of heavy weight required by athletic training can enhance existing dysfunctional patterns. For example, a non-runner whose hips are internally rotated, creating a knock-kneed stance, may have no pain at all until she starts to train for a marathon. Her movement patterns are then put to the test, and she quickly develops pain in her knees and ankles. Likewise, a man who habitually stands with an arched lower back may have no issues until he decides to get in shape and start weight-lifting. His back muscles become tighter with each repetition; soon his lower back aches constantly and the compression of his lumbar spine leads to bulging discs.

Some types of athletic training magnify our natural function of handedness, demanding a great deal from our dominant side. Many sports require throwing, hitting or kicking a ball with great force and precision, over and over again. Other disciplines, such as gymnastics and dance, require jumping, balancing and turning movements to be performed repeatedly on one side, shifting the body weight and creating imbalances in posture and strength. The sheer overuse of one side of the body is likely to lead to dysfunctional movement patterns, as well as fatigue and structural breakdown.

Those who start their athletic training at a young age may be at increased risk of developing overuse injuries because their musculoskeletal system is not fully developed. Their bones are growing quickly, and sometimes their muscles and connective tissues have not become long or strong enough to support the size of their skeleton. One in three children who compete in sports suffers pain or an injury serious enough to make them miss a game or practice. Many of these injuries will stay with them for their entire lives, even if they switch sports or stop training altogether.

In addition to children's undeveloped physical structure, another part of the problem is that they specialize in sports far too early. If you have a child, encourage them to play more than one sport. Children who play two or three sports suffer fewer injuries than those who play just one sport, because they learn how to move in varied ways depending on what sport they are playing, and give rest to overused parts of their body during each off-season.

Common sense dictates, and research has shown, that preseason conditioning, functional training, and education about proper body mechanics are effective in preventing injuries in young athletes. The emphasis at this age should be on preparing young athletes for future success and health, rather than being solely on their performance. If a quarterback needs to throw the football farther, his coach should first address how the player is throwing the ball rather than focusing on the goal of immediately increasing yardage. Most likely, his passes will get longer as his body mechanics improve.

Numerous studies have shown strong correlations between body mechanics and incidence of sports injuries. Researchers at the Sports Injuries Research Centre in Limerick, Ireland performed a two-year study with soccer players and found that back injuries, muscle strains, and knee and ankle injuries were all linked to dysfunctional postural habits such as sway back, lumbar lordosis, kyphosis, scoliosis, and lower leg misalignment. They even tested the athletes' abilities to accurately sense the alignment of their legs, and found that faulty proprioception was a predictor of ankle sprains. Other studies have had similar results, showing that misalignment of the knees and ankles leads to ankle sprains and injuries to the anterior cruciate ligament, and that athletes with poor lower back posture are more likely to suffer hamstring strains.

The fact that athletic training can enhance and create damaging patterns is not the only reason athletes suffer injuries. Athletes are also at high risk for injury because they tend to play through the pain. The desire to be tough and keep playing often prevents athletes from taking care of themselves and being proactive about their pain and injuries. Also, the stress that athletes experience during competition sends endogenous opioids coursing through their bloodstream, dulling any pain they might be experiencing. Many athletes ignore subtle warning signs of an injury, like soreness or mild pain, until it gets bad enough that it is affecting their performance. At that point, the injury has already progressed to the point at which considerable rest and retraining will be necessary to allow the injury to heal and prevent it from reoccurring.

Unless you are on the brink of winning an Olympic gold medal, playing through the pain of an injury is probably not worth it. Taking a game or a season off is difficult, but damaging your body permanently, being in chronic pain, and cutting your career short is much worse.

At this point it might seem like I am not in favor of athletic training, but quite the opposite is true. In addition to the endless physical and mental benefits that come from regular exercise, studies show that serious athletic training teaches discipline, increases life satisfaction, and improves sense of well-being. Athletes and coaches simply need to have a stronger focus on training proper movement patterns and put a higher value on injury prevention and recovery. As the saying goes, train smarter, not harder.

Clinical Somatic Education, which we'll discuss in the next chapter, has profound benefits for any type of athlete. Somatic exercises keep your muscles flexible and your joints moving freely, and are a much more effective method than static stretching for cooling down after a workout. Most importantly, Somatic exercises give you a high degree of awareness and control over your posture and movement. With regular practice of Somatic exercises, not only will you be able to use your body in an extremely precise way, you will also be able to sense when your movements are the slightest bit off, allowing you to prevent habitual misuse before it causes pain or injury.

PART FOUR
MOVING FORWARD

CHAPTER 15

Clinical Somatic Education

At this point you might be thinking, "Okay, I get it—my pain is most likely the result of the way I'm habitually using my body—so how do I stop doing damage to myself?" The simple answer to this question is that you should have in-person lessons with a Clinical Somatic Educator. The techniques involved in Clinical Somatic Education (CSE) are most effective when taught in person so that the educator can give you individualized feedback on how you are doing the movements.

If you can't find a certified educator where you live, there are a number of wonderful tools including audio recordings, books, and DVDs available to purchase online. In my practice, I offer audio recordings because I have found that they are the most effective tool when it comes to learning at home. You can lie down on the floor, close your eyes, and be guided through the movements without having to read a book or watch a video and then try to copy what you just read or saw.

The use of the word "somatic" has become quite common over the past several decades, in the realms of both holistic healthcare and Western medicine. A quick web search results in a long list of modalities ranging from psychotherapy to voice work to self-massage using balls and other props. Using the word somatic is entirely appropriate in most of these cases, as somatic is generally defined as "of, relating to, or affecting the body." However, to find educators trained in the specific method of sensory-motor education developed by Thomas Hanna, you need to look for someone who is certified in Clinical Somatic Education, Hanna Somatic Education, or Somatic Education in the tradition of Thomas Hanna.

For the sake of simplicity, we often refer to Hanna's work as "Somatics" with a capital S. While I am not going to describe the Somatic exercises here, as reading them from a book is not the best way to learn them, I do want you to understand the principles of the method and what to expect when you visit an educator for lessons.

The Principles of Clinical Somatic Education

1. Chronic musculoskeletal pain, dysfunctional posture and movement, and physical degeneration are most often caused by learned motor patterns.

Our nervous system controls our muscles, and our muscles move our skeleton around. Our body does not move in any way unless our nervous system tells it to do so. Chronic pain, chronic stress, muscle tension, postural distortions, joint degeneration, and stress fractures are most often the result of how the nervous system is functioning—how it is telling our body to stand and move.

Chronic pain, physical degeneration, and posture and movement issues can also result from things outside of voluntary nervous system control. Our genetic makeup, metabolic or immune system function, diet, activity level, and even a bacteria or virus can cause musculoskeletal pain. But if all of these possible causes have been ruled out, it is fairly safe to assume that your learned, habitual motor patterns are the cause of your issue, and they are what must be addressed in order for your function to improve.

2. Active movement on the part of the client is necessary in order to create lasting change in learned motor patterns.

CSE lessons are active on the part of the client, meaning that the client moves voluntarily during the lessons. An example of an active movement is a client lifting up their own arm. An example of a passive movement is the therapist lifting up the client's arm while the client remains relaxed. Massage, chiropractic, and most other bodywork modalities are passive.

While therapies which use only passive techniques are usually relaxing and enjoyable, the results of these therapies typically do not last more than a few days. Active movement on the part of the client is necessary in order to form new neural pathways and achieve lasting change in the functioning of the nervous system. CSE uses a combination of both passive and active movement techniques. The passive movements calm the client's nervous system and increase their internal awareness before they engage in voluntary movement, while the active movements are responsible for creating lasting change and retraining learned motor patterns.

3. The underlying cause of a problem must be addressed.

Most pain treatments, whether they be medication or a form of bodywork, address only the symptoms of the client's problem. These treatments either focus on relieving the sensation of pain or use spot work, an approach which assumes that the problem is only occurring in the area of the body where the pain is being felt. Since these treatments address only symptoms, their results typically don't last.

CSE addresses the underlying cause of pain by working with the nervous system to address full-body patterns of posture and movement. No part of the human body moves independently; with every movement, adjustments and shifts happen throughout the body that allow the movement to happen. When pain or breakdown occurs in one part of the body, is it most often a symptom of a dysfunctional full-body pattern. In order for the problem to go away for good, the entire pattern must be addressed. In every CSE lesson, the educator teaches the client movements that address the full-body patterns that are causing their pain.

4. Clinical Somatic Educators work with clients rather than on clients.

In CSE, the client is not viewed as simply a body to work on or manipulate. The client is a whole person whose thoughts, reactions, emotions and experiences have created the habitual patterns that have led to their dysfunction. The educator and the client work together in partnership throughout the series of lessons. There is verbal communication between the educator and client throughout each lesson, allowing the educator to understand what the client is experiencing and to adjust the movements based on the client's feedback.

5. Clients should be taught how to be self-sufficient instead of dependent.

Many treatments and therapies for pain are based on some sort of dependence, whether it be that the client must return on a regular basis for sessions or must continue to take medication. CSE gives people a way to take care of themselves. In fact, the method is founded upon the belief that people have the ability to and should take care of themselves instead of relying on others to maintain their health.

At every lesson, the educator teaches the client new self-care exercises which are to be practiced daily at home. The self-care exercises are slow and gentle, and most people find them to be relaxing and enjoyable. Typically, clients have between three and six hands-on lessons, though occasionally a client will have more lessons if they are working through a particularly complex issue or are in a great deal of pain. After completing a series of lessons, the client has learned enough exercises and has a deep enough understanding of the technique that they are able to continue to make progress on their own at home.

The intention of a series of lessons is to make the client their own expert; to give them the tools they need to continue to improve their self-awareness, unlearn damaging patterns, and assess themselves on a daily basis. The purpose of this process is not only to help the client regain awareness and control, but also to teach them how to guide themselves through the educational process without a practitioner.

What to expect in Clinical Somatic Education lessons

A series of lessons is a learning process, and that process is different for every client. Some people experience significant changes in their pain or functioning very quickly, while for others it takes a longer period of time. It is important to focus on the learning process rather than on the end goal.

CSE is most effective when it is approached not as a therapy but as an educational experience. You should come to lessons expecting to be a student, and should be prepared to do your homework—the self-care exercises—every day for about twenty to thirty minutes. The lessons are taught through a process designed to get you to experience in yourself how your body should feel and move. This process allows you to make long-lasting changes to your posture, movement patterns, level of muscle tension, and ability to manage stress.

CSE lessons are slow and gentle, and appropriate for those in any physical condition. You do not need to be physically fit or aerobically active, and all movements can be modified so that you can do them comfortably. You will actively participate in the lesson, consciously engaging in slow, simple movements. You will remain fully clothed, and should wear comfortable, stretchy clothing that allows for free movement.

If you are engaging in other types of treatment or therapy while going through a series of CSE lessons, you may not experience optimal results. Pain medications can interfere with your ability to sense your body accurately, so being on these medications can limit your ability to learn. Some types of bodywork may actually make your muscles tighter, and some may be confusing to your nervous system while you are attempting to make changes in learned patterns. It is generally best if you go through the relearning process without interference from passive, manipulative techniques, as well as techniques that involve intense stretching or strengthening. This holds true both during your series of lessons and afterward, when you are continuing your learning by doing the self-care exercises at home.

Your first lesson begins with an assessment in which you and your educator sit down and go over your medical history, current pain conditions, and daily lifestyle. After the verbal assessment, the educator will ask you to stand up so that they can observe your posture. The educator will gently touch the muscles in your neck, back and waist to get a sense of your muscular tension. They may observe you walking or ask you to do a few simple movements. The purpose of the assessment is for the educator to gather as much information as possible so that they can work with you in an informed way.

After your assessment, you will lie down on the Somatics table and spend forty-five to sixty minutes doing gentle movements. The educator will guide you through some of these movements with their hands, while other movements are done on your own. Some of the movements are passive, meaning that you get to completely relax and just focus on what you're feeling. These passive movements give both you and the educator a sense of your range of motion, movement patterns, and level of muscular tension. They also begin the process of relaxing the nervous system. Other movements are active, and as they are very slow and controlled, they require a great deal of mental focus. These active movements allow for the release of chronic muscular contraction and the relearning of natural, efficient movement patterns.

At the end of your lesson, you will get up and do a sitting or standing proprioceptive exercise. The proprioceptive exercises are practiced in front of a mirror, and they allow you to begin the process of changing your postural habits. By combining your internal sense of your posture with the objective view that you see in the mirror, you can learn if what you're sensing is actually correct.

Often when a client comes in for their first lesson, their proprioception is quite "off." In other words, they are sensing that their shoulders are pulled back when they are actually rounded forward, or that their hips are even when one hip is actually higher than the other. Faulty proprioception can be a significant roadblock in making changes to posture and movement. Even if a great deal of muscular release is achieved by doing Somatic exercises while lying down, our tendency is to go back into our old habits once we stand up because we instinctively want to stay balanced in gravity. It can feel wrong or uncomfortable to sit and stand in a new way. People who have tight back muscles and arched backs will feel as though they are slouching when they begin to release their back muscles. People who hold one hip higher than the other will feel off balance when their obliques are released and they begin standing and walking with their hips even. Proprioceptive training performed while sitting and standing is essential in order to maintain the release attained by Somatic exercises and prevent us from falling back into habitual patterns.

At the end of your lesson, your educator will teach you self-care exercises that you will practice at home every day. Most educators will give you a handout with written descriptions of the exercises, and in my practice I give every client an audio CD as well. I find that the audio CD is extremely helpful in guiding new clients through the exercises at an appropriate pace, and it ensures that the client is performing the exercises correctly.

Once you have learned all of the basic self-care exercises, you should practice them for twenty to thirty minutes every day. It is fine to do more than thirty minutes, but it is not necessary. The most important aspect of the self-care exercises is not how many repetitions you do, but how you do them. Practice the exercises in a quiet, private space where you will not be interrupted by family members, pets, television or background noise. You should focus all of your attention on what you're feeling as you do the movements. It is important to remember that the exercises are exploratory, so you should allow yourself to feel something new and learn something new each time you do them.

Continuing the Learning Process

By the end of a series of lessons, many clients have experienced significant reduction in their pain. However, this does not mean that their learning process is over.

We spend our entire lives developing habitual motor patterns, and for a long time they do not cause us pain. Finally one day, we begin to feel soreness or pain. The habits that are causing this discomfort have been present for many years. While it may take a relatively short time to get out of pain, the habits are still present, and it can take years to fully unlearn these damaging patterns.

While some people keep up with their Somatic exercises just enough to keep themselves out of pain, others go further with the process and continue doing the exercises for the rest of their lives. A regular Somatics practice is extremely enjoyable and rewarding. It is a process of continually discovering new sensations and new abilities in your body, and becoming aware of how wonderful your body is supposed to feel.

Regular practice of Somatic exercises is necessary not only to change deeply learned patterns, but also to release the habitual tension we build up each day. In this sense, practicing the exercises daily is much like brushing our teeth. Life keeps happening, and we keep learning new motor tasks and encountering potentially stressful situations. Just as our teeth get dirty every day, our nervous system is constantly learning new motor patterns and strengthening existing ones.

Somatic exercises have a very calming effect, a result of both decreasing muscle tension and reducing the reactivity of the nervous system. With continued regular practice of Somatic movements, you will react less to stress and experience less anxiety, thereby reducing your experience of pain.

To practice Somatic exercises on a regular basis with the intention of taking control of one's health requires a shift in thinking for many people. We've been trained to let the experts tell us how to eat, drink, exercise and medicate, and assuming the responsibility of taking care of oneself can be daunting. Developing an awareness of our internal sensations and regaining full voluntary muscular control is critical to our health because it allows us to assess and correct ourselves more quickly and effectively than if we were to wait for symptoms to appear. The human nervous system is a highly complex, extremely powerful tool, and learning how to harness its potential gives us enormous capacity to prevent pain and injury, improve the quality of our lives, and even lengthen our lives.

CHAPTER 16

Keeping Yourself in (and out of) Pain

I have seen some clients, despite their best efforts in diligently practicing Somatic exercises, prolong their pain with damaging habits. Sometimes their workout routine, stress level, attitude, and even mundane things like their footwear or desk chair are keeping them in pain. This chapter is a list, in no particular order, of habits in your daily life that might be contributing to or prolonging your pain. Consider each one individually, and don't dismiss it automatically if you don't think it applies to you. Try picking one thing to think about each day—don't overwhelm yourself by attempting to address all of your habits at once.

Move Naturally

When we are in pain, we tend to adjust our normal

movement patterns to compensate for the pain. This might mean putting more weight on the non-painful side of our body or holding parts of our body stiff as we move. These compensatory patterns quickly become learned habits, and often lead to further pain. For example, someone who has pain in their right knee will tend to put more weight on their left side, a habit which over time may lead to problems with the left hip, knee or ankle.

When you're in pain, you should try to relax and move as normally as you can. Easier said than done, but I strongly encourage you to try. This means keeping your weight distributed evenly between both feet and keeping your entire body as relaxed as possible, allowing your joints to move freely. Try not to hold any part of your body stiff, and check in with yourself periodically so that you remain aware of how you are standing and moving.

Reminding yourself to relax and move naturally will not only help prevent compensatory patterns from developing, but will also help muscular pain in particular to go away more quickly. For example, when we experience a muscle spasm, we tend to instinctively tense the spasmodic muscle and surrounding muscles even more in order to splint the injury and prevent movement that could worsen the pain. Generally, preventing movement of a spasmodic muscle will only serve to keep it tight. By imagining that you are not in pain and letting yourself move naturally—but slowly and gently, if you are experiencing a spasm—you will be allowing the muscle to gently contract and release as you move, and you will gradually regain voluntary control.

Keep Moving

We know that there are countless benefits to getting regular exercise. It improves cardiovascular fitness, muscle strength, bone density, brain function and mental health, and reduces the risk of developing cancer and heart disease. It shouldn't come as a big surprise that we can add preventing and alleviating chronic pain to the list.

A great deal of research has shown that regular exercise reduces rates of chronic pain, and there are a number of reasons why. Regular movement is necessary to maintain flexibility of muscles and connective tissues. Exercise improves circulation, which speeds up the healing process and keeps joints healthy by increasing blood flow in and around them. Exercise also increases proprioceptive awareness and improves posture, and creates the opportunity for you to improve your body mechanics. If you sit all day at your job and get no exercise, you'll likely spend little time thinking about the way that you stand and move. Even if you have an active job, it is difficult to think about improving your body mechanics when you are focused on a task at work. Exercise gives you the opportunity to get out of habitual postural and movement patterns you might have developed on the job. Lastly, exercise triggers the release of endorphins and has even been shown to increase confidence. By putting you in a positive state of mind, exercise decreases anxiety and negative thought patterns, thereby reducing the unpleasantness of pain.

But here's the catch: what if exercise worsens your pain? Or what if your exercise of choice seems to have caused your pain or injury in the first place? If you find yourself in this situation, start by moving slowly and gently. Try doing a different type of exercise so that you will be less likely to use your body in the habitual way that caused your pain. Going for a slow walk, practicing Tai Chi, or swimming can all be good low-impact options. Don't worry about the fact that you're not doing your normal high-intensity workout. The most important thing is to find a way to keep moving.

Move Smarter, Not Harder

As a result of habitual muscular tension and stress, many of us use more force than necessary to perform the simplest of everyday activities. We grip the steering wheel as we drive to work and keep our whole upper body tense as we work at our computers. All of this unnecessary tension adds to and can be the cause of our pain.

We even overuse our muscles when we exercise. Many athletes hold unnecessary tension throughout their bodies when they move. Not only can this result in injury, but it is quite inefficient as far as energy usage. All of those tight muscles are constantly burning fuel unnecessarily.

Try an experiment: go through your day using as little muscular effort as possible to perform every movement, from brushing your teeth and preparing breakfast to running on the treadmill and lifting heavy objects. You'll be forced to use good body mechanics instead of muscular force to carry out the movements. You'll reduce your resting level of muscle tension and feel more relaxed overall. You may be surprised at how impactful this simple experiment can be.

Stop Fixating on Your Pain

When you're in pain, it is difficult to think about anything else. Pain is generally so unpleasant and potentially dangerous that when we are feeling it, our number one instinct is to find a way to make it stop.

While it is hard to avoid, fixating on your pain often leads to stress and anxiety. These in turn increase your level of muscle tension, trigger reflexive postural patterns, and worsen your perception of pain. It can be quite challenging, but I encourage you to take deep breaths, relax and do your best to forget about the pain—even if it's just for a few moments at a time.

Fixating on your pain often leads to damaging behavioral habits as well, such as subconsciously popping and cracking joints. Sudden movement of a joint often results in temporary relief from the pain, which is why we instinctively do it. But repeated popping and cracking can actually increase joint inflammation and overstretch soft tissues, ultimately increasing your pain.

For example, people with TMJ disorders may feel their jaw moving out of alignment due to tight muscles and connective tissues creating an imbalance in the joint. Some people with TMJ disorders develop the habit of popping the joint throughout the day because the popping gives them a brief sense of relief. Often they pop the joint without even thinking about it and are unaware of how often they do it. This habit alone can prolong the pain that initially began due to stress or a dysfunctional movement pattern. While doing Somatic exercises should reduce the urge to pop the joint, all the Somatic exercises in the world may not relieve the pain if they continue aggravating the joint tissues by popping the joint.

My simple advice to clients who have damaging habits like popping and cracking a joint or doing a deep stretch of a tight muscle is to "stop messing with it." Every time you have the urge, just stop, take a deep breath and relax. Better yet, you can substitute your habit with a Somatic exercise that will relieve your tension without aggravating the joint or overstretching the tight muscle.

Stop Being Tough

We touched on this subject in the chapter "Training Pain," but it's important to note here that athletes are not the only ones guilty of hurting themselves by toughing it out. Many people keep quiet about their pain because they don't want to be viewed as weak or they worry that their family and friends are sick of hearing them complain. Unfortunately, the result of ignoring your pain is that you may be allowing the problem to get worse.

Please stop ignoring or hiding your pain. Acknowledge it, and resolve to find a way to address it. It takes a tough, intelligent person to know when to rest and take care of their body. Remember, this is the only body you get for your entire life—don't abuse it.

Improve Your Proprioception

Improving your proprioceptive awareness is the first step in creating change in your posture and movement. If your proprioception—the way you sense your body in space—is off, you may feel as though you are standing and sitting straight when in fact you aren't. Following are a few simple exercises you can do to begin improving your proprioception.

First exercise: Stand normally, arms hanging by your sides, and just relax—don't try to stand with perfect posture. Wear fitted clothing and no shoes. Have someone take photos of you from the front, back and both sides. While you're standing there, and before you look at the photos, close your eyes and have your friend ask you the following questions:

Do you feel like your weight is more on the balls of your feet or your heels? Does it feel like there is there more weight on one foot than the other?

Do you feel like your knees are locked and pushed back, fairly straight, or slightly bent? Does one knee feel different than the other?

Do you feel like you are arching your back and sticking out your belly, or tucking your pelvis under and contracting your abdominals?

Does it feel like one hip is higher than the other?

Do you feel that your shoulders are rounding forward, fairly neutral, or being pulled back so that you are sticking out your chest?

Does it feel like one shoulder is higher than the other?

Do you feel like your head is sitting right on top of your spine, pulled back, or jutting forward?

Imagine a straight line running up the side of your body and going through these five points: ankle, knee, hip, shoulder and ear. Is this actually a straight line? Are any of these body parts forward or behind the line?

Once you have answered all these questions, you can open your eyes and look at your photos. You'll find out if what you see in the photos matches up with what you were feeling. You may want to ask your friend what they see, because your friend's interpretation of the photos will be more objective than yours.

Second exercise: Sit on a stool or chair with a flat seat, and move forward so that you're not leaning back in the seat. Let your thighs be parallel to the ground or sloping downward (so that your knees are lower than your hips), and make sure your ankles are directly under your knees or in front of your knees. Close your eyes, and very slowly and gently roll your hips forward and backward until you find a place in the middle where you feel like you are sitting straight up and down. Ask your friend to take a photo of you in this position. Then look at the photo, and find out if what you see in the photo matches up with what you were feeling.

Third exercise: Set an alarm on your phone or watch to go off every ten minutes throughout the day. Pick the happiest, least annoying alarm sound you can. Each time the alarm goes off, take a moment to close your eyes, take a deep breath, and let go of all the muscular tension you're holding on to subconsciously. Notice where in your body you tend to hold tension. Afterward, see how long you can stay relaxed as you go back to your normal activities. You'll likely be surprised at not only how much tension you're holding on to subconsciously, but also at how quickly you're able to train yourself to stay relaxed.

Switch Sides

We've talked about the effects of handedness on habitual motor patterns, and how simply using the sides of your body in different ways can lead to pain and structural damage. Exploring the ways that you use the sides of your body differently will help you become more aware of your learned patterns and allow you to change them. To begin this process, try the following activities. One by one, perform each movement with the side that you typically use, then use your other side.

-Brush your teeth
-Brush your hair
-Rest your weight on one side
-Balance on one leg
-Carry a bag on your shoulder
-Use a computer mouse
-Kick a ball
-Bend forward and pick up a small, light object

At first, you may feel that you are literally incapable of performing these simple tasks with your non-dominant side. When you feel like this, slow down and analyze the movement. How are you moving, what adjustments are you making, and what muscles are you engaging in order to carry out this task with your dominant side? Once you have a sense of the body mechanics involved in the movement, try doing it with your non-dominant side. Go back and forth from side to side until the movement starts to feel natural on your non-dominant side. This process will increase your awareness and control of your non-dominant side and train you to have more balanced body mechanics.

Improve the Ergonomics of Your Daily Life

Ergonomics, the practice of designing and arranging things so that people can use them efficiently and safely, is typically talked about in the context of our work environment. However, you should consider the ergonomics of your home and other spaces that you use on a regular basis as well. The ways that we adapt to our physical surroundings and to the equipment and furniture that we use play a large role in developing dysfunctional motor patterns. Consider how you adapt to your surroundings while doing the following activities.

When driving, adjust your seat so that the back and head rest are supportive. You should be able to sit straight up and down with your shoulders relaxed and not rounded forward. Try to use both arms equally to control the steering wheel. Check in with yourself every few minutes so that you can adjust your posture and release any unnecessary muscle tension.

If you spend a lot of time talking on the phone, you should use a headset or keep the phone on speaker. Holding a phone up to your ear requires you to keep your arm in a bent position and tilt your head to the side. Neck pain is a common complaint among folks who spend a lot of time on the phone.

Whether you use a computer at work, at home or both, take some time to create an ideal setup for yourself. Your computer screen should be at eye level, not below, so that you can look straight ahead rather than downward while you're working. Your screen should be directly in front of your chair so that you don't have to twist or turn in order to work. The screen should be an appropriate distance away from you so that you don't have to strain your eyes or lean forward in order to see what you're working on. Remember, you can zoom in on documents and web sites instead of craning your neck forward. Your wrists should be in a neutral, relaxed angle when typing; this means that your keyboard should be at the height of your elbows or slightly above your elbows. Your chair should have a high enough back so that you feel fully supported and do not need to use any effort to sit up straight. The seat of your chair should be flat rather than tipped backward. While working at your computer, you should feel that you are in a relaxed, neutral position. Check in with yourself periodically throughout the day and remind yourself of what that relaxed, neutral position feels like.

When you're at home, consider the ergonomics of the areas where you spend the most time. For example, many of us spend time every day relaxing on the couch, either watching television, reading or using electronics. Notice the way you sit or lie on the couch. Do you tend to lean to one side or the other? If so, try to switch sides, or find a comfortable neutral position in which you can relax. When watching television, make sure you can look straight ahead at the screen rather than having to turn your head to see. Also consider the couch itself: the higher the back, the more supportive it will be and the easier it will be for you to sit up straight without straining your neck. You can use pillows behind your back and neck to create the ideal supportive setup for yourself.

Aside from your workstation, the place where you spend the most time is your bed, so consider your mattress and your sleeping position. Your mattress should be firm enough to be supportive but soft enough to allow your hips and shoulders to sink in a bit. Whatever position you sleep in, the most important thing is that your spine should be in a straight, neutral position. This means that if you sleep on your back, you should not be using a pillow. In order to maintain a straight spine while on your back, your head should be resting directly on the mattress. Lying on your back and using a pillow is equivalent to standing with your head jutting forward eight hours a day. If you have back pain, consider sleeping on your back with a pillow under your knees; this will take the pressure off your lower back and allow your spine to rest in a neutral position.

If you sleep on your side, use a pillow that allows your neck to be straight. Formed pillows that provide shaped support for your neck and head are wonderful for side sleeping. The firmness of the mattress is quite important for side sleepers; your hips and shoulders must be able to sink down enough that your spine remains straight.

If you sleep on your stomach, I strongly encourage you to start sleeping on your back or your side. Stomach sleeping is terrible for your neck, as it requires that your neck be turned to one side or the other. Lying on your stomach also creates tightness and compression in your lower back. It may take some time to train yourself to sleep on your back or your side, but it will be worth it in the long run.

Choose Proper Footwear

We evolved wearing no shoes at all, and our feet are structured to comfortably hold our body weight with no additional support. However, it might not feel like that if you are accustomed to wearing thick-soled sneakers, arch support inserts, or high heels. This is because your movement patterns and the resting level of tension in the muscles of your feet and legs have adapted to your footwear.

Consider the fit of your shoes. If they are too tight or restrictive, you may experience bunion pain or cramping in the muscles of your feet. If your shoes are too loose, the way that you walk and run will be affected and you may experience hip, knee or ankle problems. Your shoes should be roomy enough that your feet truly feel comfortable, yet fitted enough that your feet aren't moving around as you walk and run.

The soles of your shoes should be flexible. You should be able to hold your shoe by the heel and toe and fold it in half. A flexible sole allows the muscles of your feet to do their job, and allows you to move in a way that is most similar to being barefoot.

Some of you may not like to hear this, but you knew it was coming: don't wear high heels. Any shoe that has a raised heel shifts an unnatural amount of weight onto the ball of the foot, especially onto the big toe joint. For this reason, high heels are one of the main causes of bunion pain. Raised heels also keep the Achilles tendon and the muscles of the foot and calf in a shortened state for long periods of time, leading to chronic tightness, muscle cramps, and plantar fasciitis.

The soles of your shoes should be as thin as you are comfortable wearing. This is most often an issue with sneakers. Whether you are wearing thick-soled sneakers for running, walking, or just around during the day, having extra cushioning under the heel allows you to strike the ground harder than you would if you were barefoot. Heel-striking puts unnecessary strain and pressure on your feet, ankles and knees, and contributes to poor body mechanics.

That being said, we evolved to walk and run on dirt and grass rather than concrete. If you are walking or running long distances on concrete, you may find that you are more comfortable wearing sneakers with some cushioning. Ultimately, the amount of cushioning in your sneakers is not the most important thing—it's your walking and running form. If you do wear sneakers with thick soles, please make sure that they are flexible, and consider having your running form analyzed to ensure that you are not heel-striking.

Lastly, I recommend varying your footwear from day to day, especially if you spend a lot of time on your feet. This will help prevent you from developing poor body mechanics as a result of your shoes. Remember, your natural movement patterns should not be altered by the shoes you wear.

Take some time to go through your closet and take stock of your footwear. Find the shoes that are comfortably fitted with thin, flexible soles and no raised heels; these are the shoes you should be wearing the majority of the time.

Reduce Stress

We've talked about how stress causes and worsens your pain: by increasing muscular tension, triggering postural reflexes, and altering your perception of pain. If you haven't already, now I would like you to start thinking about ways that you can reduce stress in your life.

Magazines offer us "Ten Ways to Reduce Stress," suggesting taking bubble baths, listening to relaxing music, and breathing deeply. While these activities will temporarily reduce your stress, the underlying cause of your stress that must be addressed is your thought patterns. Do you perceive situations to be stressful when in reality they aren't? Do you spend a great deal of time worrying and creating unnecessary stress in your mind?

Research shows that by and large it is not experiences themselves but the way that we perceive and process them which determines the effects that stress has on our motor patterns and pain conditions. In a study of over 48,000 Swedish military recruits between the ages of eighteen and twenty-four, over 5,000 of them already had back problems—and the strongest predictor of their back pain was their ability to manage stress. Another study showed that among migraine sufferers, headaches could be predicted not just by stressful occurrences but also by the test subjects' interpretation of the events and their ability to cope with the stress.

Two people in identical situations can perceive and react to the situations in very different ways. Can you think of someone you know who is always stressed out? Catastrophes occur for him on a daily basis, and he is always worrying or freaking out about something. More than likely, he does not encounter more stressful situations than the average person. But does he have more stress in his life? Absolutely—because he creates it.

We are the only beings on the planet who have the ability to change our thought patterns and choose how we interpret situations. If we perceive a situation to be stressful, our stress response will be triggered. We also predetermine how we react by worrying about potentially stressful situations ahead of time. We may not feel that we can choose how we react because our responses and thought patterns have become habitual—much like we feel that we can't change our posture and movement patterns because they have become so deeply learned that they are outside our voluntary control.

When you find that you are feeling stressed out, ask yourself: is your or someone else's life or health being threatened in some way? If not, then there is generally no benefit to you allowing your stress response to be activated. The stress that you and the people around you experience creates an unpleasant working or living environment, negative expectations, impatience, poor communication, and a decrease in productivity.

Begin to notice what happens when you experience stress. Does your posture change? Do your muscles get tense? If you're in pain, does your pain get worse? Does your pulse race? Do your thoughts become fixated on the stressful situation? Does your stress affect the way you react to non-stressful things in your life? Do you take the stress out on your family, friends or co-workers?

Once you have begun to notice your habitual reactions to stress, you can begin to change them. Take a deep breath into your lower belly, hold it for a few seconds, and exhale as slowly as you can. Analyze your situation and look at it objectively. Can you find a way to remain relaxed and deal with the situation? If you can, you'll find that not only is your stress reduced, but the stress of the other people involved is reduced as well. Stress is contagious! You have the ability to turn a potentially stressful situation into a neutral and even positive experience for everyone involved just by modifying your reaction.

It takes time to retrain your habitual thought patterns and reactions, but just like changing your habitual motor patterns, it's worth the time and effort. Try it today: notice one potentially stressful situation that you encounter, take a deep breath, and try to relax and turn it into a positive experience.

Expect to Get Better

We know from our earlier discussion of the placebo effect that if we expect to get better, we generally will. Unfortunately, the opposite can also occur: if we expect to get worse, we generally will. When you're in pain, it can be quite difficult to believe that you will get better. But finding a way to have a positive attitude is one of the best things you can do for yourself.

The increase in pain resulting from having negative expectations is referred to as *nocebo hyperalgesia*, and research has shown how this effect occurs at a neurobiological level. Brain imaging studies show increased activation of a pain pathway known as the medial pain system when subjects expect that a stimulus will be painful. So it is important to understand that having a negative expectation doesn't just mean that people are reporting more pain—it means that they are actually experiencing more pain.

Researchers have found that they can predict which surgical patients will experience greater postoperative pain based on presurgical assessment using the Pain Catastrophizing Scale. The scale measures how fixated the patients are on their pain, to what extent they magnify their pain and expect that it will get worse, and their feelings of helplessness. The more that patients catastrophize about their pain before the surgery, the more pain they experience afterward. Researchers are now investigating whether or not they can reduce patients' postoperative pain by modifying their attitude before surgery.

Over the course of our lives, we develop habitual ways of thinking just as we develop habitual ways of standing and moving. It is easy for us to get stuck in our thought patterns, and can be very difficult to get objective feedback on how we think and even more difficult to take the feedback. But as a good friend of mine says, "Don't believe everything you think." Just because you think something doesn't mean that it is true.

It feels safe to stay in habitual patterns, whether they be ways of thinking or ways of standing and moving. It can also feel like it is impossible to change our thought patterns because they have become automatic. Like changing our motor patterns, it takes patience and time to change our ways of thinking. If you find yourself thinking negatively about your pain, stop yourself and try to think about your situation in the opposite way. Instead of "My back is just going to get worse and worse. I'll never be able to hike again," practice telling yourself "My back is going to get better! This pain is going to go away and I'm so excited to go hiking again!"

With practice, positive thinking will become easier and even habitual. And remember, positive thinking won't just improve your attitude—it will actually reduce your experience of pain on a neurobiological level. It will also change your behavior. If you think that you can get better, you will be more diligent about practicing self-care exercises daily because you'll believe that they will work.

Don't Expect Change to Happen Overnight

Our society demands fast results and miracle cures. But if you've ever tried any diet or exercise plan which promises guaranteed results in a short amount of time, you've probably learned from experience that lasting change rarely comes easily or quickly. This is especially true when it comes to getting out of pain and changing deeply learned motor patterns. You've spent your entire life developing the habitual patterns that are now causing your pain, so it is unreasonable to expect that these patterns can be changed and that your pain will go away forever in a matter of days or weeks. Embarking on a process of changing habitual patterns is like beginning a journey without knowing exactly where it will take you or when you'll arrive.

Like any learning process, you'll get out of it what you

put into it. Practicing Somatic exercises every day for twenty to thirty minutes is ideal, though there is no harm in practicing for longer periods of time. Just keep in mind that your nervous system and the bones and tissues of your body can only change so fast. Doing more will not necessarily get you better or faster results, and in general, slow change is best. Your progress will have more to do with how you practice the exercises and how well you are able to integrate what you've learned from the exercises into your daily life.

You may find it helpful to keep a journal or log of how you feel on a day to day basis. Each day you can note whether or not you did your exercises and rate your pain on a scale of 0 to 10. You can also make notes about what might be affecting your pain that day, such as activities you did, your sleep pattern, and your mood. Keeping a log like this can help you track your progress, can help you notice patterns in your pain, and can help you remember your experiences accurately.

Keep in mind that your improvement will probably not follow a straight upward path. There will be days when you feel great and other days when you don't. You may be pain-free for months and then have an old pain suddenly return or a new pain emerge. Making changes in your posture and movement, even when they are changes for the better, can cause some soreness or discomfort simply because you are using your body in an unfamiliar way. Going through a process of change is rarely a smooth journey—you'll encounter some bumps in the road, and they are usually nothing to worry about.

Don't Wait

The longer you let your pain persist, the more damage you can do to your body and the more sensitized your nervous system can become. The best thing you can do for yourself is to stop ignoring your pain and find a way to address it in a constructive way. Don't wait—do it today!

CHAPTER 17

Next Steps

So, how do we move forward in our effort to reduce the amount of pain that we are living with? Simply understanding how to change our learned motor patterns may not be enough to make a significant impact on the prevalence of pain and physical degeneration in our society. Many of us expect to be chronically stressed, uncomfortable and in pain. It's almost as if we want to suffer. In order for us to get out of pain, we need to shift our attitude; we must expect to improve instead of decline with age. We must understand that we are supposed to feel wonderful and comfortable in our bodies.

Next, we must accept responsibility for our health and be willing to do the work to keep ourselves healthy. Many doctors and patients would rather pursue treatment that offers an easy fix, even if that fix is only temporary and comes with side effects, than put time and energy into improving health for the long term. The reality is that there are very few quick fixes or miracle cures when it comes to our health. We need to want to be self-sufficient and to appreciate how wonderful it is to be able to rely on ourselves instead of others.

Many people don't get motivated to take care of themselves until their health begins to decline. Most pain and disease conditions exist on a spectrum, and must get to a certain threshold in order to be diagnosed and treated. By that time the condition has already progressed to the point at which a great deal of time and treatment will be required to alleviate or eliminate it. We need to understand that it is much simpler and easier to take a preventative, proactive approach to our health than to wait until something bad happens. We accept that we need to practice healthy habits like eating well and exercising in order to prevent obesity, diabetes and heart disease. The next step is to accept that we need to maintain our sensory-motor awareness and practice Somatic exercises throughout our lives in order to prevent pain, injury and musculoskeletal degeneration.

CSE must be taught at an early age and made accessible to everyone. Both Thomas Hanna and F.M. Alexander believed that the best application of somatic education would be to teach it in schools so that children could learn the skills they need to take care of themselves for the rest of their lives. In addition, health insurance plans must start covering CSE so that it is affordable for everyone. CSE should appeal to health insurance companies because they could save a great deal of money on medications and surgeries for pain by covering preventative care. However, if we sit around and wait for schools and health insurance companies to start offering CSE, it will never happen; we must demand it.

The potential reward for taking care of our musculoskeletal health is huge. Besides reducing the $600 billion per year drain on the U.S. economy, we have the opportunity to greatly improve our quality of life. CSE gives us the ability to prevent, alleviate and eliminate our own pain; remain active and productive; and lengthen our own lives. Not only has it effectively given me a new body, it has also calmed my nervous system and greatly reduced my reactions to stress. I hope you move forward with the knowledge you gained in this book and seek out your nearest certified educator. Clinical Somatic Education has profoundly improved my life, and I know it can do the same for you.

Acknowledgments

To Patrick Flanagan and Philip Warren, for their thoughtful reading and insightful feedback.

To my parents, for always encouraging my creativity.

To my co-workers, for the constant support, motivation and inspiration.

And to my husband, for his support, patience and entertainment throughout the writing process.

Illustration Credits

Illustration 1: The Structure of a Neuron
Adapted from 3drenderings/123rf.com

Illustration 2: The Structure of the Brain
Adapted from Alila/123rf.com

Illustration 3: The Somatosensory and Motor Cortices
Adapted from Designua/123rf.com

Illustration 4: Hyperkyphosis
Undrey/123rf.com

Illustration 5: Typical Computer Posture
Innovatedcaptures/123rf.com

Illustration 6: Natural Spinal Curvature
Adapted from Vonuk/123rf.com

Illustration 7: Personality and Posture
Zurijeta/123rf.com

References

CHAPTER 1: The Problem of Pain

A new hope for back pain sufferers? (2012, May 6). CBS News. Retrieved from http://www.cbsnews.com/news/a-new-hope-for-back-pain-sufferers

American Cancer Society. *Cancer Treatment & Survivorship: Facts and Figures, 2014-2015.* Retrieved November 4, 2014 from http://www.cancer.org/acs/groups/content/@research/documents/document/acspc-042801.pdf

American Heart Association. (2011). Heart Disease and Stroke Statistics---2011 Update: A Report From the American Heart Association. *Circulation, 2011, 123,* e18-e209. doi:10.1161/CIR.0b013e3182009701

American Pain Foundation. (2006, May). *Voices of Chronic Pain Survey.* Conducted by David Michaelson & Company, LLC.

Apkarian, A.V. et al. (2004, November 17). Chronic Back Pain Is Associated with Decreased Prefrontal and Thalamic Gray Matter Density. *The Journal of Neuroscience, 24*(46), 10410-10415.

Apkarian, A.V. et al. (2004, March). Chronic pain patients are impaired on an emotional decision-making task. *PAIN 108* (1-2), 129–136.

Bair, M.J., MD, MS; Robinson, R.L., MS; Katon, W., MD; & Kroenke, K., MD. (2003, November 10). Depression and Pain

Comorbidity: A Literature Review. *Archives of Internal Medicine, 163*(20), 2433-2445. doi:10.1001/archinte.163.20.2433

Baliki, M.N.; Geha, P.Y.; Apkarian, A.V.; & Chialvo, D.R. (2008, February 6). Beyond Feeling: Chronic Pain Hurts the Brain, Disrupting the Default-Mode Network Dynamics. *The Journal of Neuroscience, 28*(6), 1398-1403. doi:10.1523/JNEUROSCI.4123-07.2008

Centers for Disease Control and Prevention. (2011). *Heart Disease and Stroke Prevention: Addressing the Nation's Leading Killers---At a Glance 2011.* Retrieved from http://www.cdc.gov/chronicdisease/resources/publications/aag/pdf/2011/heart-disease-and-stroke-aag-2011.pdf

Centers for Disease Control and Prevention. (2014). *National Diabetes Statistics Report: Estimates of Diabetes and Its Burden in the United States.* Atlanta, GA: U.S. Department of Health and Human Services.

Centers for Disease Control and Prevention. (2005). Prevalence and Most Common Causes of Disability Among Adults---United States, 2005. *Morbidity and Mortality Weekly Report, 58*(16), 421-426.

Centers for Disease Control and Prevention. (2011, November 4). Vital Signs: Overdoses of Prescription Opioid Pain Relievers---United States, 1999-2008. *Morbidity and Mortality Weekly Report, 60*(43), 1487-1492.

Committee on Advancing Pain Research, Care, and Education; Institute of Medicine of the National Academies. (2011, June 29). *Relieving Pain in America: A Blueprint for Transforming Prevention, Care, Education and Research.* Washington, D.C.: The National Academies Press.

Deyo, R.A., MD, MPH et al. (2010, April 7). Trends, Major Medical Complications, and Charges Associated With

Surgery for Lumbar Spinal Stenosis in Older Adults. *The Journal of the American Medical Association, 303*(13), 1259-1265. doi:10.1001/jama.2010.338

Deyo, R.A., MD, MPH; Rainville, J., MD; & Kent, D.L., MD. (1992). What can the history and physical examination tell us about low back pain? *The Journal of the American Medical Association, 268*(6), 760–765.

Farina, K.L., PhD. (2012). The Economics of Cancer Care in the United States. *American Journal of Managed Care, 2012.*

Grachev, I.D.; Fredrickson, B.E.; & Apkarian, A.V. (2000, December 15). Abnormal brain chemistry in chronic back pain: an in vivo proton magnetic resonance spectroscopy study. *PAIN 89*(1), 7–18.

Lucas, A.J. (2012, November 22). Failed back surgery syndrome: whose failure? Time to discard a redundant term. *British Journal of Pain, 6,* 162. doi:10.1177/2049463712466517

Martin, B.I., MPH et al. (2008). Expenditures and Health Status Among Adults With Back and Neck Problems. *The Journal of the American Medical Association, 299*(6), 656-664. doi:10.1001/jama.299.6.656

Mazer-Amirshahi, M., PharmD, MD; Mullins, P.M., MA; Rasooly, I.; van den Anker, J. MD, PhD; & Pines, J.M., MD, MBA, MSCE. (2014). Rising Opioid Prescribing in Adult U.S. Emergency Department Visits: 2001-2010. *Academic Emergency Medicine, 21*(3), 236-243. doi:10.1111/acem.12328

National Centers for Health Statistics. (2006). Chartbook on Trends in the Health of Americans. *Health, United States.*

National Sleep Foundation. (2001, March). *2001 "Sleep in America" Poll.* Conducted by WB&A Market Research.

Nguyen, T.H., MD, PhD; Randolph, D.C., MD, MPH; Talmage, J., MD; Succop, P., PhD; & Travis, R., MD. (2011, February 15). Long-term Outcomes of Lumbar Fusion Among Workers' Compensation Subjects: A Historical Cohort Study. *Spine, 36*(4), 320-331. doi:10.1097/BRS.0b013e3181ccc220

Painkillers fuel growth in drug addiction. (2011, January). *Harvard Mental Health Letter.* Retrieved from http://www.health.harvard.edu/newsletters/ Harvard_Mental_Health_Letter/2011/January/painkillers-fuel-growth-in-drug-addiction

Paulozzi, L., MD, MPH. *The Prescription Drug Overdose Epidemic and the Role of PDMPs in Stopping It.* PDMP Center of Excellence. Retrieved November 4, 2014 from http://www.pdmpexcellence.org/sites/all/pdfs/ Paulozzi_12_2010.pdf

Prescription Pain Medicines—An Addictive Path? (2007). *NIH Medline Plus, 2*(4), 22.

Research!America. (2003). *Americans Talk About Pain: A Survey Among Adults Nationwide.* Conducted by Peter D. Hart Research Associates. Retrieved from https://www.researchamerica.org/uploads/poll2003pain.pdf

Substance Abuse and Mental Health Services Administration. (2011). *Results from the 2010 National Survey on Drug Use and Health: Summary of National Findings.* Rockville, MD: Substance Abuse and Mental Health Services Administration.

Suddath, Claire. (2011, March 11). Living with Pain. *Time.*

Tavernise, S. (2013, January 25). F.D.A. Likely to Add Limits on Painkillers. *The New York Times,* p. A1.

The National Center on Addiction and Substance Abuse at Columbia University. (2012, June). *Addiction Medicine: Closing the Gap between Science and Practice.* Retrieved from http://www.casacolumbia.org/addiction-research/reports/addiction-medicine

The National Center on Addiction and Substance Abuse at Columbia University. (2000, April). *Missed Opportunity: National Survey of Primary Care Physicians and Patients on Substance Abuse.* Conducted by the Survey Research Laboratory, University of Illinois at Chicago.

The National Center on Addiction and Substance Abuse at Columbia University. (1998, June). *Under the Rug: Substance Abuse and the Mature Woman.* Retrieved from http://www.casacolumbia.org/addictionresearch/reports/under-the-rug-substance-abuse-mature-woman

Tsang, A. et al. (2008, October). Common Chronic Pain Conditions in Developed and Developing Countries: Gender and Age Differences and Comorbidity With Depression-Anxiety Disorders. *The Journal of Pain, 9*(10), 883-891. doi:10.1016/j.jpain.2008.05.005

CHAPTER 2: Understanding Pain

Apkarian, A.V. (2010). Human Brain Imaging Studies of Chronic Pain. *Translational Pain Research: From Mouse to Man.* Editors: Kruger, L. & Light, A.R. Boca Raton, FL: CRC Press.

Apkarian, A.V.; Bushnell, M.C.; Treede, R.D.; & Zubieta, J.K. (2005, August). Human brain mechanisms of pain perception and regulation in health and disease. *European Journal of Pain, 9*(4), 463-484.

Arnstein, P.M. (1997, June). The neuroplastic phenomenon: a physiologic link between chronic pain and learning. *Journal of Neuroscience Nursing, 29*(3), 179-186.

Bear, M.F.; Connors, B.W.; & Paradiso, M.A. (2007). *Neuroscience: Exploring the Brain* (3rd ed). Baltimore, MD: Lippincott Williams & Wilkins.

Borgens, R.B.; Shi, R. (2000, January). Immediate recovery from spinal cord injury through molecular repair of nerve membranes with polyethylene glycol. *The FASEB Journal, 14*(1), 27-35.

Braun, C.A. & Anderson, C.M, PhD. (2007) *Pathophysiology: functional alterations in human health.* Baltimore, MD: Lippincott Williams & Wilkins.

Coderre, T.J.; Katz, J.; Vaccarino, A.L.; & Melzack, R. (1993, March). Contribution of central neuroplasticity to pathological pain: review of clinical and experimental evidence. *PAIN, 52*(3), 259-295.

Correll, G.E.; Maleki, J.; Gracely, E.J.; Muir, J.; & Harbut, R.E. (2004, September). Subanesthetic Ketamine Infusion Therapy: A Retrospective Analysis of a Novel Therapeutic Approach to Complex Regional Pain Syndrome. *Pain Medicine, 5*(3), 263-275.

De Mos, M. et al. (2007, May). The incidence of complex regional pain syndrome: A population-based study. *PAIN, 129(1-2),* 12-20. doi:10.1016/j.pain.2006.09.008

Egger, G., PhD, MPH. (2012). In Search of a Germ Theory Equivalent for Chronic Disease. *Preventing Chronic Disease, 9,* 110301. doi:10.5888/pcd9.110301

Eriksson, P.S. et al. (1998). Neurogenesis in the adult human hippocampus. *Nature Medicine, 4,* 1313-1317. doi:10.1038/3305

Ferrero-Miliani, L.; Nielsen, O.H.; Andersen, P.S.; & Girardin, S.E. (2007, February). Chronic inflammation: importance of NOD2 and NALP3 in interleukin-1beta generation. *Clinical*

& *Experimental Immunology, 147*(2), 227-235.

Hunter, P. (2012, September 10). The inflammation theory of disease. *EMBO reports, 13,* 968-970. doi:10.1038/embor.2012.142

IASP Taxonomy. Retrieved October 11, 2014, from International Association for the Study of Pain (http://www.iasp-pain.org/Taxonomy?navItemNumber=576).

Juhan, D. (2003). *Job's Body: A Handbook for Bodywork* (3rd ed.). Barrytown, NY: Barrytown/Station Hill Press, Inc.

Kidd, B.L. & Urban, L.A. (2001). Mechanisms of Inflammatory Pain. *British Journal of Anaesthesia, 87*(1), 3-11.

Kiefer, R., MD; Rohr, P., MD; Ploppa, A., MD; Altemeyer, K., MD; & Schwartzman, R.J., MD. (2007). Complete Recovery From Intractable Complex Regional Pain Syndrome, CRPS-Type I, Following Anesthetic Ketamine and Midazolam. *Pain Practice, 7*(2), 147-150.

Lu, H. et al. (2011, January). Macrophages recruited via CCR2 produce insulin-like growth factor-1 to repair acute skeletal muscle injury. *The FASEB Journal, 25*(1), 358-369.

Marinus, J. et al. (2011). Clinical features and pathophysiology of complex regional pain syndrome. *Lancet Neural, 10,* 637-648.

McMurray, G.A., PhD. (1950, November). Experimental Study of a Case of Insensitivity to Pain. *AMA Archives of Neurology & Psychiatry, 64*(5), 650-667. doi:10.1001/archneurpsyc.1950.02310290046005

Melzack, R. & Wall, P.D. (2008). *The Challenge of Pain* (2nd ed.). London, England: Penguin Books, Ltd.

Mense, S., MD. (2003, December). The Pathogenesis of Muscle Pain. *Current Pain and Headache Reports, 7*(6), 419-425.

Mense, S., MD. (2000). *Pathophysiology of muscle pain.* Pain in Europe III. EFIC 2000, Nice, France, September 26-29, 2000. Retrieved from http://www.painstudy.ru/pe3/muscle_pain.htm

Petersen-Felix, S. & Curatolo, M. (2002). Neuroplasticity – an important factor in acute and chronic pain. *Swiss Medical Weekly, 132,* 273–278.

Price, D.D. (2000, June 9). Psychological and Neural Mechanisms of the Affective Dimension of Pain. *Science, 288*(5472), 1769-1772. doi:10.1126/science.288.5472.1769

Rainville, P.; Duncan, G.H.; Price, D.D.; Carrier, B.; & Bushnell, M.C. (1997, August 15). Pain Affect Encoded in Human Anterior Cingulate But Not Somatosensory Cortex. *Science, 177,* 968-971.

Roth, S.M. (2006, January 23). Why does lactic acid build up in muscles? And why does it cause soreness? *Scientific American,* Ask the Experts. Retrieved from http://www.scientificamerican.com/article/why-does-lactic-acid-buil/

Safari, A.; Khaledi, A.A.; & Vojdani, M. (2011, February). Congenital Insensitivity to Pain with Anhidrosis (CIPA): A Case Report. *Iranian Red Crescent Medical Journal, 13*(2), 134-138.

Salomons, T.V.; Johnstone, T.; Backonja, M.; & Davidson, R.J. (2004, August 11). Perceived Controllability Modulates the Neural Response to Pain. *The Journal of Neuroscience, 24*(32), 7199-7203. doi:10.1523/JNEUROSCI.1315-04.2004

Sandroni, P.; Benrud-Larson, L.M.; McClelland, R.L.; & Low, P.A. (2003, May). *PAIN, 103*(1-2), 199-207.

Sapolsky, R.M. (2004). *Why Zebras Don't Get Ulcers: The Acclaimed Guide to Stress, Stress-Related Diseases, and Coping* (3rd ed.). New York, NY: Holt Paperbacks/Henry Holt and Company, LLC.

Schmidt, C.E. & Leach, J.B. (2003). Neural tissue engineering: strategies for repair and regeneration. *Annual Review of Biomedical Engineering, 5,* 293-347.

Seifert, F. & Maihofner, C. (2011). Functional and structural imaging of pain-induced neuroplasticity. *Current Opinion in Anaesthesiology, 24*(5), 515-523. doi:10.1097/ACO.0b013e32834a1079

Stackhouse, S.K.; Reisman, D.S.; & Binder-Macleod, S.A. (2001, December). Challenging the Role of pH in Skeletal Muscle Fatigue. *Physical Therapy, 81*(12), 1897-1903.

Tinazzi, M. et al. (2000, December 15). Neuroplastic Changes Related to Pain Occur at Multiple Levels of the Human Somatosensory System: A Somatosensory-Evoked Potentials Study in Patients with Cervical Radicular Pain. *The Journal of Neuroscience, 20*(24), 9277-9283.

Vithoulkas, G. & Carlino, S. (2010, February). The "continuum" of a unified theory of disease. *Medical Science Monitor, 16*(2), SR7-15.

Wilkinson, P.R. (2001). Neurophysiology of pain Part I: Mechanisms of pain in the peripheral nervous system. *CPD Anaesthesia, 3*(3), 103-08.

CHAPTER 3: Why Stress Makes It Worse

2010 Fibromyalgia Diagnostic Criteria – Excerpt. Retrieved October 12, 2014, from American College of Rheumatology (http://www.rheumatology.org/Practice/Clinical/ Classification/Fibromyalgia/2010_Fibromyalgia_ Diagnostic_Criteria_-_Excerpt/).

Asmundson, G., PhD; Coons, M.J., BA; Taylor, S., PhD; & Katz, J., PhD. (2002, December). PTSD and the Experience of Pain: Research and Clinical Implications of Shared Vulnerability and Mutual Maintenance Models. *The Canadian Journal of Psychiatry, 47,* 930-937.

Bear, M.F.; Connors, B.W.; & Paradiso, M.A. (2007). *Neuroscience: Exploring the Brain* (3rd ed). Baltimore, MD: Lippincott Williams & Wilkins.

Bondy, B. et al. (2003, March 15). Substance P serum levels are increased in major depression: preliminary results. *Biological Psychiatry, 53*(6), 538-542.

Brown, E.S., MD, PhD; Rush, A.J., MD; & McEwen, B.S., PhD. (1999). Hippocampal Remodeling and Damage by Corticosteroids: Implications for Mood Disorders. *Neuropsychopharmacology, 21*(4), 474-484.

Burgmer, M. et al. (2012, May). Cerebral mechanisms of experimental hyperalgesia in fibromyalgia. *European Journal of Pain, 16*(5), 636-647.

Cohen, H. et al. (2002, August). Prevalence of post-traumatic stress disorder in fibromyalgia patients: overlapping syndromes or post-traumatic fibromyalgia syndrome? *Seminars in Arthritis & Rheumatism, 32*(1), 38-50.

Colloca, L. & Benedetti, F. (2007, October). Nocebo hyperalgesia: how anxiety is turned into pain. *Current Opinion in Anaesthesiology, 20*(5), 435-439.

Defrin, R. et al. (2008). Quantitative testing of pain perception in subjects with PTSD: Implications for the mechanism of the coexistence between PTSD and chronic pain. *PAIN, 138*(2), 450-459.

Depression and Pain. (2004). *Harvard Mental Health Letter.* Retrieved October 15, 2014 from Harvard Health Publications (http://www.health.harvard.edu/newsweek/Depression_and_pain.htm).

Grachev, I.D.; Frederickson, B.E.; & Apkarian, A.V. (2002). Brain chemistry reflects dual states of pain and anxiety in chronic low back pain. *Journal of Neural Transmission, 109,* 1309-1334. doi:10.1007/s00702-002-0722-7

Grachev, I.D.; Fredrickson, B.E.; & Apkarian, A.V. (2001). Dissociating anxiety from pain: mapping the neuronal marker N-acetyl aspartate to perception distinguishes closely interrelated characteristics of chronic pain. *Molecular Psychiatry, 6,* 256-260.

Juhan, D. (2003). *Job's Body: A Handbook for Bodywork* (3rd ed.). Barrytown, NY: Barrytown/Station Hill Press, Inc.

Keefe, F.J. Et al. (2001, April). Pain and emotion: new research directions. *Journal of Clinical Psychology, 57*(4), 587-607.

Keltner, J.R. et al. (2006, April 19). Isolating the Modulatory Effect of Expectation on Pain Transmission: A Functional Magnetic Resonance Imaging Study. *The Journal of Neuroscience, 26*(16), 4437-4443.

Kling, M.A.; Coleman, V.H.; & Schulkin, J. (2009). Glucocorticoid inhibition in the treatment of depression: can we think outside the endocrine hypothalamus? *Depression and Anxiety, 26*(7), 641-649. doi:10.1002/da/20546

Kroenke, K. et al. (2013). Association between anxiety, health-related quality of life and functional impairment in primary care patients with chronic pain. *General Hospital Psychiatry, 35*(4), 359-365.

Libman, B.S., MD. The Most Common Autoimmune Disease: Rheumatoid Arthritis. Retrieved October 12, 2014, from http://www.med.uvm.edu/downloads/CMS_Libman_Autoimmune_051810.pdf

McEwen, B.S. (2005, May). Glucocorticoids, depression, and mood disorders: structural remodeling in the brain. *Metabolism, 54*(5 Suppl 1), 20-23.

McEwen, B.S. (1999). Stress and hippocampal plasticity. *Annual Review of Neuroscience, 22,* 105-122.

McIntyre, C.K. & Roozendaal, B. (2007). Adrenal Stress Hormones and Enhanced Memory for Emotionally Arousing Experiences. *Neural Plasticity and Memory: From Genes to Brain Imaging.* Editor: Bermudez-Rattoni, F. Boca Raton, FL: CRC Press.

Mengshoel, A.M. & Heggen, K. (2004, January 7). Recovery from fibromyalgia – previous patients' own experiences. *Disability and Rehabilitation, 26*(1), 46-53.

Murphy, B.E.P. (1991, May). Steroids and depression. *The Journal of Steroid Biochemistry and Molecular Biology, 38*(5), 537-559.

Otis, J.D., PhD; Keane, T.M., PhD; & Kerns, R.D., PhD. (2003). An examination of the relationship between chronic pain and post-traumatic stress disorder. *Journal of Rehabilitation Research and Development, 40*(5), 397-406.

Prevalence of fibromyalgia. Retrieved October 12, 2014, from National Fibromyalgia Association (http://www.fmaware.org/prevalence.html).

Roth, R.S.; Geisser, M.E.; & Bates, R. (2008, July). The relation of post-traumatic stress symptoms to depression and pain in patients with accident-related chronic pain. *The Journal of Pain, 9*(7), 588-596. doi:10.1016/j.jpain.2008.01.333

Salomons, T.V.; Johnstone, T.; Backonja, M.; & Davidson, R.J. (2004, August 11). Perceived Controllability Modulates the Neural Response to Pain. *The Journal of Neuroscience, 24*(32), 7199-7203. doi:10.1523/JNEUROSCI.1315-04.2004

Sapolsky, R.M. (2003, November). Stress and Plasticity in the Limbic System. *Neurochemical Research, 28*(11), 1735-1742.

Sapolsky, R.M. (2004). *Why Zebras Don't Get Ulcers: The Acclaimed Guide to Stress, Stress-Related Diseases, and Coping* (3rd ed.). New York, NY: Holt Paperbacks/Henry Holt and Company, LLC.

Schwarz, M.J., MD & Ackenheil, M., MD. (2002, March). The role of substance P in depression: therapeutic implications. *Dialogues in Clinical Neuroscience, 4*(1), 21-29.

Sharp, T.J. & Harvey, A.G. (2001, August). Chronic pain and posttraumatic stress disorder: mutual maintenance? *Clinical Psychology Review, 21*(6), 857-877.

Watanabe, Y.; Gould, E.; & McEwen, B.S. (1992, August 21). Stress induces atrophy of apical dendrites of hippocampal CA3 pyramidal neurons. *Brain Research, 588*(2), 341-345. doi:10.1016/0006-8993(92)91597-8

What is fibromyalgia? Retrieved October 12, 2014, from The American Fibromyalgia Syndrome Association, Inc (http://www.afsafund.org/fibromyalgia.html).

What is fibromyalgia? Retrieved October 12, 2014, from National Institute of Arthritis and Musculoskeletal and Skin Diseases (http://www.niams.nih.gov/Health_Info/Fibromyalgia/fibromyalgia_ff.asp).

Yuen, E.Y. et al. (2009, August 18). Acute stress enhances glutamatergic transmission in prefrontal cortex and facilitates working memory. *Proceedings of the National Academy of Sciences, 106*(33), 14075-14079. doi:10.1073/pnas.0906791106

CHAPTER 4: Natural Pain Relief

Afghanistan: Chronology of opium through history. (2004, August 2). Retrieved October 13, 2014 from IRIN (http://www.irinnews.org/indepthmain.aspx? InDepthId=21&ReportId=63040).

Assefi, N.P. et al. (2005). A Randomized Clinical Trial of Acupuncture Compared with Sham Acupuncture in Fibromyalgia. *Annals of Internal Medicine, 143,* 10-19.

Associated Press. (2012, August 9). *Runner finishes on broken leg.* Retrieved October 13, 2014 from ESPN (http://espn.go.com/olympics/summer/2012/trackandfield/ story/_/id/8251820/2012-london-olympics-us-runner-manteo-mitchell-finishes-4x400-meter-relay-broken-leg).

Bear, M.F.; Connors, B.W.; & Paradiso, M.A. (2007). *Neuroscience: Exploring the Brain* (3rd ed). Baltimore, MD: Lippincott Williams & Wilkins.

Beecher, H.K. (1956, August 25). Relationship of significance of wound to pain experienced. *The Journal of the American Medical Association, 161*(17), 1609-1613. doi:10.1001/jama.1956.02970170005002

Boecker, H. et al. (2008). The Runner's High, Opioidergic Mechanisms in the Human Brain. *Cerebral Cortex, 18*(11), 2523-2531.

Clement-Jones, V. et al. (1980, November 1). Increased beta-endorphin but not met-enkephalin levels in human cerebrospinal fluid after acupuncture for recurrent pain. *The Lancet, 2*(8201), 946-949.

Cloud, J. (2011, March 11). Beyond Drugs. *TIME.* Retrieved from http://content.time.com/time/specials/packages/printout/ 0,29239,2053382_2055260,00.html

Colt, E.W.; Wardlaw, S.L.; & Frantz, A.G. (1981, April 6). The effect of running on plasma beta-endorphin. *Life Sciences, 28*(14), 1637-40.

De Craen, A.J.; Kaptchuk, T.J.; Tijssen, J.G.; & Kleijnen, J. (1999, October). Placebos and placebo effects in medicine: historical overview. *Journal of the Royal Society of Medicine, 92*(10), 511-515.

DosSantos, M.F. et al. (2012, November 2). Immediate effects of tDCS on the micro-opioid system of a chronic pain patient. *Frontiers in Psychiatry, 3,* 93. doi:10.3389/fpsyt.2012.00093

Goddard, G.; Karibe, H.; McNeill, C.; & Villafuerte, E. (2002). Acupuncture and sham acupuncture reduce muscle pain in myofascial pain patients. *Journal of Orofacial Pain, 16*(1), 71-76.

Guillemin, R. et al. (1977, September). !b-endorphin and adrenocorticotropin are secreted concomitantly by the pituitary gland. *Science, 197*(4311), 1367-1369.

Han, J. (2004). Acupuncture and endorphins. *Neuroscience Letters, 361,* 258-261.

Levine, J.D.; Gordon, N.C.; & Fields, H.L. (1978, September 23). The mechanism of placebo analgesia. *The Lancet, 2*(8091), 654-657.

Linde, K. et al. (2009, January 21). Acupuncture for migraine prophylaxis. *Cochrane Database of System Reviews, 1,* CD001218.

Melzack, R. & Wall, P.D. (2008). *The Challenge of Pain* (2nd ed.). London, England: Penguin Books, Ltd.

Moffet, H.H. (2009, March). Sham acupuncture may be as efficacious as true acupuncture: a systematic review of clinical trials. *Journal of Alternative and Complementary Medicine,*

15(3), 213-216. doi:10.1089/acm.2008.0356

Opium throughout history. *Frontline.* Retrieved October 13, 2014 from PBS (http://www.pbs.org/wgbh/pages/frontline/shows/heroin/etc/history.html).

Pert, C.B. & Snyder, S.H. (1973, March 9). Opiate receptor: demonstration in nervous tissue. *Science, 179*(4077), 1011-1014. doi:10.1126/science.179.4077.1011

Petrovic, P.; Kalso, E.; Petersson, K.M.; & Ingvar, M. (2002, March 1). Placebo and Opioid Analgesia---Imaging a Shared Neuronal Network. *Science Magazine, 295,* 1737-1740.

Rudgley, R. (1999). *The Lost Civilizations of the Stone Age.* New York: The Free Press.

Sapolsky, R.M. (2004). *Why Zebras Don't Get Ulcers: The Acclaimed Guide to Stress, Stress-Related Diseases, and Coping* (3rd ed.). New York, NY: Holt Paperbacks/Henry Holt and Company, LLC.

Simon, E.J.; Hiller, J.M.; & Edelman, I. (1973, July). Stereospecific binding of the potent narcotic analgesic (3H) Etorphine to rat-brain homogenate. *Proceedings of the National Academies of Sciences, 70*(7), 1947-1949. doi:10.1073/pnas.70.7.1947

Stix, G. (2014, March 3). Can Acupuncture Reverse Killer Inflammation? *Talking Back.* Retrieved October 22, 2014 from Scientific American (http://blogs.scientificamerican.com/talking-back/2014/03/03/can-acupuncture-reverse-killer-inflammation/).

Terenius, L. (1973). Stereospecific interaction between narcotic analgesics and a synaptic plasma membrane fraction of rat cerebral cortex. *Acta Pharmacologica et Toxicologica (Copenh), 32*(3), 317-320. doi:10.1111/j.1600-0773.1973.tb01477.x

Torres-Rosas, R. et al. (2014, March). Dopamine mediates vagal modulation of the immune system by electroacupuncture. *Nature Medicine, 20*(3), 291-295. doi:10.1038/nm.3479

Valance, A.K. (2006). Something out of nothing: the placebo effect. *Advances in Psychiatric Treatment, 12*, 287-296.

What is the history of opioid addiction in the United States? Retrieved October 13, 2014 from National Institute on Drug Abuse (http://www.drugabuse.gov/international/question-2-what-history-opioid-addiction-in-united-states#joseph).

White, A. & Ernst, E. (2004). A brief history of acupuncture. *Rheumatology, 43*(5), 662-663. doi:10.1093/rheumatology/keg005

Woods, J. *The Discovery of Endorphins.* Retrieved October 13, 2014 from National Alliance of Methadone Advocates (http://www.methadone.org/library/woods_1994_endorphin.html).

Wu, J. (1996). A Short History of Acupuncture. *The Journal of Alternative and Complementary Medicine, 2*(1), 19-21. doi:10.1089/acm.1996.2.19

Yilmaz, P. et al. (2010, November). Brain correlates of stress-induced analgesia. *PAIN, 151*(2), 522-529. doi:10.1016/j.pain.2010.08.016

Young, D. (2007, April 15). *Scientists Examine Pain Relief and Addiction.* Retrieved from AJHP News (http://www.ashp.org/menu/News/PharmacyNews/NewsArticle.aspx?id=2509).

CHAPTER 5: Developing Habitual Patterns

Adams, J.A. (1987). Historical Review and Appraisal of Research on the Learning, Retention, and Transfer of Human Motor Skills. *Psychological Bulletin, 101*(1), 41-74.

Attwell, P.J.E.; Cooke, S.F.; & Yeo, C.H. (2002, June 13). Cerebellar Function in Consolidation of a Motor Memory. *Neuron, 34,* 1011-1020.

Bear, M.F.; Connors, B.W.; & Paradiso, M.A. (2007). *Neuroscience: Exploring the Brain* (3rd ed). Baltimore, MD: Lippincott Williams & Wilkins.

Berlucchi, G. & Buchtel, H.A. (2009, January). Neuronal Plasticity: historical roots and evolution of meaning. *Experimental Brain Research, 192*(3), 307-319.

Dekaban, A.S., (1978, October). Changes in brain weights during the span of human life: relation of brain weights to body heights and body weights. *Annals of Neurology, 4*(4), 345-356.

Doyon, J. & Benali, H. (2005). Reorganization and plasticity in the adult brain during learning of motor skills. *Current Opinion in Neurobiology, 15,* 161-167.

Eden, S. (2013, January 22). *Stroke of madness.* Retrieved October 14, 2014 from ESPN The Magazine (http://espn.go.com/golf/story/_/id/8865487/tiger-woods-reinvents-golf-swing-third-time-career-espn-magazine).

Feldenkrais, M. (2005). *Body & Mature Behavior.* Berkeley, CA: Frog Books/ North Atlantic Books.

Hanna, T. (2004). *Somatics: Reawakening the Mind's Control of Movement, Flexibility, and Health.* Cambridge, MA: De Capo Press. Hanna, T. (1993). *The Body of Life.* Rochester, VT: Healing Arts Press.

Hill, L.B. (1934). A Quarter Century of Delayed Recall. *The Pedagogical Seminary and Journal of Genetic Psychology,*

44(1), 231-238. doi:10.1080/08856559.1934.10532492

Houk, J. (2010). Voluntary Movement: Control, Learning and Memory. *Encyclopedia of Behavioral Neuroscience, 3,* 455-458.

James, W. (1890). Chapter IV: Habit. *The Principles of Psychology,* Volume 1. Retrieved from Classics in the History of Psychology, http://psychclassics.yorku.ca/James/Principles/prin4.htm

Juhan, D. (2003). *Job's Body: A Handbook for Bodywork* (3rd ed.). Barrytown, NY: Barrytown/Station Hill Press, Inc.

Liu, J.; Thornell, L.; & Pedrosa-Domellof, F. (2003, February). Muscle Spindles in the Deep Muscles of the Human Neck: A Morphological and Immunocytochemical Study. *Journal of Histochemistry & Cytochemistry, 51*(2), 175-186.

Ma, L. et al. (2010, March 8). Changes in Regional Activity Are Accompanied with Changes in Inter-Regional Connectivity during Four Weeks Motor Learning. *Brain Research, 1318C,* 64-76. doi:10.1016/j.brainres.2009.12.073

Melzack, R. & Wall, P.D. (2008). *The Challenge of Pain* (2nd ed.). London, England: Penguin Books, Ltd.

Newmark, T., MD. (2012, October). Cases in Visualization for Improved Athletic Performance. *Psychiatric Annals, 42*(10), 385-387.

Packard, M.G. & Knowlton, B.J. (2002). Learning and memory functions of the Basal Ganglia. *Annual Review of Neuroscience, 25,* 563-593.

Roland, P.E.; Larsen, B.; Lassen, N.A.; & Skinhoj, E. (1980, January). Supplementary motor area and other cortical areas in organization of voluntary movements in man. *Journal of Neurophysiology, 43*(1), 118-136.

Santos, M.J.; Kanekar, N.; & Aruin, A.S. (2010, June). The role of anticipatory postural adjustments in compensatory control of posture: 1. Electromyographic analysis. *Journal of Electromyography & Kinesiology, 20*(3), 388-397. doi:10.1016/j.jelekin.2009.06.006

Shadmehr, R. & Holcomb, H.H. (1997, August 8). Neural Correlates of Motor Memory Consolidation. *Science Magazine, 277,* 821-825.

Shaffer, D.R. & Kipp, K. (2009). *Developmental Psychology: Childhood and Adolescence* (8th ed). Belmont, CA: Wadsworth Publishing.

Shutoh, F.; Ohki, M.; Kitazwa, H.; Itohara, S.; & Nagao, S. (2006, May 12). Memory trace of motor learning shifts transsynaptically from cerebellar cortex to nuclei for consolidation. *Neuroscience,* 139(2), 767-777.

Stefan, K. et al. (2005, October 12). Formation of a Motor Memory by Action Observation. *The Journal of Neuroscience, 25*(41), 9339-9346.

Strata, P. (2009, December 1). David Marr's theory of cerebellar learning: 40 years later. *The Journal of Physiology, 587,* 5519-5520. doi:10.1113/jphysiol.2009.180307

Tiger Woods Statistics. (2013, December 23). Retrieved October 14, 2014 from Statistic Brain (http://www.statisticbrain.com/tiger-woods-statistics/).

Webster, M.A. (2012). Evolving concepts of sensory adaptation. *F1000 Biol Reports, 4,* 21. doi:10.3410/B4-21

Wolpert, D.M.; Ghahramani, Z.; & Flanagan, J.R. (2001, November). Perspectives and problems in motor learning. *TRENDS in Cognitive Sciences, 5*(11), 487-494.

CHAPTER 6: When Our Patterns Cause Pain

Alfredson, H. & Lorentzon, R. (2002, February). Chronic tendon pain: no signs of chemical inflammation but high concentrations of the neurotransmitter glutamate. Implications for treatment? *Current Drug Targets, 3*(1), 43-54.

Headache disorders, Fact sheet No.277. (2012, October). Retrieved October 15, 2014 from World Health Organization (http://www.who.int/mediacentre/factsheets/fs277/en/).

IHS Classification ICHD-II: Introduction to the Classification. Retrieved October 15, 2014 from International Headache Society Classification (http://www.ihs-classification.org/en/01_einleitung/02_einleitung/).

Juhan, D. (2003). *Job's Body: A Handbook for Bodywork* (3rd ed.). Barrytown, NY: Barrytown/Station Hill Press, Inc.

Malanga, G.A.; Nadler, S.F.; Bowen, J.E.; Feinberg, J.H.; & Hyman, G.S. (2004). Sports Medicine. *Physical Medicine and Rehabilitation: Principles and Practice, Volume 1.* Edited by DeLisa, J.A.; Gans, B.M.; & Walsh, N.E. Baltimore, MD: Lippincott Williams & Wilkins.

National Headache Foundation Fact Sheet. Retrieved October 15, 2014 from http://www.health-exchange.net/pdfdb/headfactEng.pdf

Sainsbury, P. & Gibson, J.G. (1954). Symptoms of Anxiety and Tension and the Accompanying Physiological Changes in the Muscular System. *Journal of Neurology, Neurosurgery & Psychiatry, 17,* 216-224.

Schwellnus, M.P. (2009). Cause of Exercise Associated Muscle Cramps (EAMC) –altered neuromuscular control, dehydration or electrolyte depletion? *British Journal of Sports Medicine,*

43, 401-408. doi:10.1136/bjsm.2008.050401

Tension-Type Headache. Retrieved October 15, 2014 from National Headache Foundation (http://www.headaches.org/education/Headache_Topic_Sheets/Tension-Type_Headache).

Werner, R. (2008). *A Massage Therapist's Guide to Pathology* (4th ed.). Baltimore, MD: Lippincott Williams & Wilkins.

CHAPTER 7: Why Conventional Treatments Sometimes Work, but Often Don't

Avela, J.; Kyrolainen, H.; & Komi, P.V. (1999, April 1). Altered reflex sensitivity after repeated and prolonged passive muscle stretching. *Journal of Applied Physiology, 86*(4), 1283-1291.

Bear, M.F.; Connors, B.W.; & Paradiso, M.A. (2007). *Neuroscience: Exploring the Brain* (3rd ed). Baltimore, MD: Lippincott Williams & Wilkins.

Calvert, R.N. (2014, April 24). *Pages from History: Swedish Massage.* Retrieved October 15, 2014 from Massage Magazine (http://www.massagemag.com/magazine-2002-issue100-history100-24-26).

Cherkin, D.C., PhD; Deyo, R.A., MD, MPH; Battié, M., PhD, RPT; Street, J., MN, CPNP; & Barlow, W., PhD. (1998, October 8). A Comparison of Physical Therapy, Chiropractic Manipulation, and Provision of an Educational Booklet for the Treatment of Patients with Low Back Pain. *New England Journal of Medicine, 339,* 1021-1029. doi:10.1056/NEJM199810083391502

Coombes, B.K., MPhty; Bisset, L., PhD; & Vicenzino, B. PhD. (2010, November 20). Efficacy and safety of corticosteroid injections and other injections for management of tendinopathy: a systematic review of randomized controlled trials. *The Lancet, 376*(9754), 1751-1767.

Ernst, E., MD, PhD, FRCP. (2007, July). Adverse effects of spinal manipulation: a systematic review. *Journal of the Royal Society of Medicine, 100*(7), 330-338.

Ernst, E., MD, PhD, FRCP. (2002, October). Chiropractic Care: Attempting a Risk-Benefit Analysis. *American Journal of Public Health, 92*(10), 1603-1604.

Fritz, J.M., PhD, PT, ATC; Cleland, J.A., PhD, DPT, FAAOMPT; Speckman, M.; Brennan, G.P., PhD, PT; Hunter, S.J., MS, PT, OCS. (2008, July 15). Physical Therapy for Acute Low Back Pain: Associations With Subsequent Healthcare Costs. *Spine, 33*(16), 1800-1805. doi:10.1097/BRS.0b013e31817bd853

Gelhorn, A.C., MD; Chan, L., MD; Martin, B., MPH; & Friedly, J., MD. (2012, April 20). Management Patterns in Acute Low Back Pain: The Role of Physical Therapy. *Spine (Phila Pa 1976), 37*(9), 775-782.

Gergley, J.C. (2013, April). Acute effect of passive static stretching on lower-body strength in moderately trained men. *The Journal of Strength & Conditioning Research, 27*(4), 973-977.

Gouveia, L.O.; Castanho, P.; & Ferreira, J.J. (2009, May 15). Safety of chiropractic interventions: a systematic review. *Spine (Phila Pa 1976), 34*(11), E405-413.

Hernandez-Reif, M. et al. (2004, July). Breast cancer patients have improved immune and neuroendocrine functions following massage therapy. *Journal of Psychosomatic Research, 57*(1), 45-52.

History of Chiropractic Care. Retrieved October 15, 2014 from American Chiropractic Association (http://www.acatoday.org/level3_css.cfm?T1ID-13&T2ID=61&T3ID=149).

Juhan, D. (2003). *Job's Body: A Handbook for Bodywork* (3rd ed.). Barrytown, NY: Barrytown/Station Hill Press, Inc.

Marks, L. (2005). *Bridging the Great Divide: Touching Our Most Basic Humanity.* Retrieved October 15, 2014 from http://www.healingheartpower.com/article1.html

Massage Therapy for Health Purposes: What You Need To Know. Retrieved October 15, 2014 from National Center for Complementary and Alternative Medicine (http://nccam.nih.gov/health/massage/ massageintroduction.htm).

Radcliff, K., MD et al. (2013, February 15). Epidural Steroid Injections Are Associated With Less Improvement in Patients With Lumbar Spinal Stenosis: A Subgroup Analysis of the Spine Patient Outcomes Research Trial. *Spine, 38*(4), 279-291.

Schleip, R. (2003, January). Fascial plasticity – a new neurobiological explanation: Part 1. *Journal of Bodywork and Movement Therapies, 7*(1), 11-19.

Simic, L.; Sarabon, N.; & Markovic, G. (2013, March). Does pre-exercise static stretching inhibit maximal muscular performance? A meta-analytical review. *Scandinavian Journal of Medicine & Science in Sports, 23*(2), 131-148.

Tsao, J.C.I. (2007, June). Effectiveness of Massage Therapy for Chronic, Non-malignant Pain: A Review. *Evidence-based Complementary and Alternative Medicine, 4*(2), 165-179.

Wellens, F., Bsc, pht, RCAMPT. (2010). *The traditional mechanistic paradigm in the teaching and practice of manual therapy: Time for a reality check.* Retrieved October 16, 2014 from PhysioAxis (http://www.physioaxis.ca/realitycheck.pdf).

Zwanger, M., MD, MBA. *Narcotic Abuse.* Edited by Dryden-Edwards, R., MD. Retrieved October 15, 2014 from eMedicineHealth (http://www.emedicinehealth.com/narcotic_abuse/article_em.htm).

CHAPTER 8: A Century of Exploration

Alexander, F.M. (2001). *The Use of the Self.* London, England: Orion Books Ltd.

Behnke, E.A. (1990). *Friends Passing: Thomas Hanna (1928-1990).* Retrieved October 14, 2014 from Somatic Systems Institute (http://somatics.org/library/bea-passing.html).

Feldenkrais, M. (2005). *Body & Mature Behavior.* Berkeley, CA: Frog Books/ North Atlantic Books.

Feldenkrais, M. (1942). *Practical Unarmed Combat.* London, England: Frederick Warne & Co., Ltd.

Gelb, M.J. (1996). *Body Learning: An Introduction to the Alexander Technique* (2nd ed). New York, NY: Henry Holt and Company, LLC.

Hanna, T. (2004). *Somatics: Reawakening the Mind's Control of Movement, Flexibility, and Health.* Cambridge, MA: De Capo Press.

Hanna, T. (1993). *The Body of Life.* Rochester, VT: Healing Arts Press.

Huebner, M. (2010). The Life and Teachings of Elsa Gindler. *Rosen Method International Journal, 3*(1), 17-21.

Klinkenberg, N. (2002). The Encounter Between Moshe Feldenkrais and Heinrich Jacoby. *Feldenkrais und Jacoby – Eine Begegnung, Volume I.* Retrieved October 14, 2014 from http://davidzemach-bersin.com/2012/09/the- encounter-between-moshe-feldenkrais-and-heinrich-jacoby/

Melville, T. *Eutony*. Retrieved October 14, 2014 from Thinking Through the Body (http://www.thinkbody.co.uk/seminars/Eutony-Gerda-Alexander.pdf).

Milz, H., MD. (1991). A Conversation with Thomas Hanna, PhD. *Somatics: Magazine-Journal of the Bodily Arts and Sciences, VIII*(2), 50-56.

Mower, M. (1990, November). In Memory of Thomas Hanna. *Massage, Nov/Dec 1990*, 73.

Pinchas, R.L.B. (1986). "The Energy Is in the Bones": Eutony's Gerda Alexander. *Yoga Journal, Jan/Feb 1986*, 21-24.

Weaver, J. (2004). The Influence of Elsa Gindler-Ancestor of Sensory Awareness. *The United States Association of Body Psychotherapy Journal, 3*(1), 22-26.

CHAPTER 9: Stress and Posture

Blouin, J.S.; Siegmund, G.P.; & Inglis, J.T. (2007, April 1). Interaction between acoustic startle and habituated neck postural responses in seated subjects. *Journal of Applied Physiology, 102*(4), 1574-1586. doi:10.1152/japplphysiol.00703.2006

Eaton, R.C. (1984). *Neural Mechanisms of Startle Behavior*. New York, NY: Springer.

Fowler, K. & Kravitz, L. PhD. *The Perils of Poor Posture*. Retrieved October 16, 2014 from IDEA Health & Fitness Association (www.ideafit.com/fitness-library/the-perils-of-poor-posture).

Guimond, S. & Massrieh, W. (2012, May 18). Intricate Correlation between Body Posture, Personality Trait and Incidence of Body Pain: A Cross-Referential Study Report. *PloS ONE*,

7(5), e37450. doi:10.1371/journal.pone/0037450

Hanna, T. (2004). *Somatics: Reawakening the Mind's Control of Movement, Flexibility, and Health.* Cambridge, MA: De Capo Press.

Hazlett, R.L.; McLeod, D.R.; & Hoehn-Saric, R. (1994, March). Muscle tension in generalized anxiety disorder: Elevated muscle tonus or agitated movement? *Psychophysiology, 31*(2), 189-195.

Juhan, D. (2003). *Job's Body: A Handbook for Bodywork* (3rd ed.). Barrytown, NY: Barrytown/Station Hill Press, Inc.

Kapandji, I.A., MD. (2008). *The Physiology of the Joints, Volume III* (6th ed). London, England: Churchill Livingstone.

Lundberg, U. et al. (1994, December). Psychophysiological stress and emg activity of the trapezius muscle. *International Journal of Behavioral Medicine, 1*(4), 354-370.

Malmo, R.B.; Shagass, C.; & Davis, J.F. (1951). Electromyographic studies of muscular tension in psychiatric patients under stress. *Journal of Clinical & Experimental Psychopathology, 12,* 45-66.

Malmo, R.B. (1975). *On Emotions, Needs, and our Archaic Brain.* Austin, TX: Holt, Rinehart and Winston, Inc.

Rideout, V.J., MA; Foehr, U.G., PhD; & Roberts, D.F., PhD. (2010, January). *Generation M2: Media in the Lives of 8- to 18-Year-Olds.* Menlo Park, CA: The Henry J. Kaiser Family Foundation.

Sainsbury, P. & Gibson, J.G. (1954, August). Symptoms of Anxiety and Tension and the Accompanying Physiological Changes in the Muscular System. *Journal of Neurology, Neurosurgery, & Psychiatry, 17*(3), 216-224.

CHAPTER 10: Injury, Handedness and Scoliosis

Bear, M.F.; Connors, B.W.; & Paradiso, M.A. (2007). *Neuroscience: Exploring the Brain* (3rd ed). Baltimore, MD: Lippincott Williams & Wilkins.

Blouin, J.S.; Corbeil, P.; & Teasdale, N. (2003, October 17). Postural Stability is altered by the stimulation of pain but not warm receptors in humans. *BMC Musculoskeletal Disorders, 4*, 23.

Carter, O.D. & Haynes, S.G. (1987). Prevalence Rates for Scoliosis in US Adults: Results from the First National Health and Nutrition Examination Survey. *The International Journal of Epidemiology, 16*(4), 537-544.

Erwin, W.D.; Dickson, J.H.; & Harrington, P.R. (1980, December). Clinical review of patients with broken Harrington rods. *The Journal of Bone & Joint Surgery-American volume, 62*(8), 1302-1307.

Ha, K.Y.; Lee, J.S.; & Kim, K.W. (2008, May 15). Degeneration of Sacroiliac Joint After Instrumented Lumbar or Lumbosacral Fusion: a Prospective Cohort Study over Five-year Follow-up. *Spine, 33*(11), 1192-1198.

Hanna, T. (2004). *Somatics: Reawakening the Mind's Control of Movement, Flexibility, and Health.* Cambridge, MA: De Capo Press.

Hanna, T. (1993).*The Body of Life.* Rochester, VT: Healing Arts Press.

Information and Support. Retrieved October 16, 2014 from National Scoliosis Foundation (http://www.scoliosis.org/info.php).

Johnston, D.W.; Nicholls, M.E.R.; Shah, M.; & Shields, M.A.

(2009, May). Nature's experiment? Handedness and early childhood development. *Demography, 46*(2), 281-301. doi:10.1353/dem.0.0053

Levin, D.A.; Hale, J.J.; & Bendo, J.A. (2007). Adjacent segment degeneration following spinal fusion for degenerative disc disease. *Bulletin of the NYU Hospital for Joint Diseases, 65*(1), 29-36.

Kebaish, K.M.; Neubauer, P.R.; Voros, G.D.; Khoshnevisan, M.A.; & Skolasky, R.L. (2011, April 20). Scoliosis in adults aged forty years and older: prevalence and relationship to age, race, and gender. *Spine (Phila PA 1976), 36*(9), 731-736.

Reamy, B.V. & Slakey, J.B. (2001, July 1). Adolescent Idiopathic Scoliosis: Review and Current Concepts. *American Family Physician, 64*(1), 111-117.

Shah, S.A., MD. (2009). *What is Scoliosis?* Retrieved October 16, 2014 from Nemours (http://www.nemours.org/content/dam/nemours/wwwv2/filebox/service/medical/spinescoliosis/scoliosisguide.pdf).

Uomini, N.T. (2009, October). The prehistory of handedness: Archaeological data and comparative ethology. *Journal of Human Evolution, 57*(4), 411-419.

Weiss, H.R. & Goodall, D. (2008, August 5). Rate of complications in scoliosis surgery – a systematic review of the Pub Med literature. *Scoliosis, 3,* 9. doi:10.1186/1748-7161-3-9

Wong, G.T.C.; Yuen, V.M.; Chow, B.F.; & Irwin, M.G. (2007, October). Persistent pain in patients following scoliosis surgery. *European Spine Journal, 16*(10), 1551-1556.

CHAPTER 11: The Daily Grind

Britnell, S.J. et al. (2005, May). Postural Health in Women: The Role of Physiotherapy. *Journal of obstetrics and gynaecology Canada, 27*(5), 493-510.

Straker, L.M.; O'Sullivan, P.B.; Smith, A.J.; Perry, M.C. (2007). Computer Use and Habitual Spinal Posture in Australian Adolescents. *Public Health Reports, 122*(5), 634-643.

CHAPTER 12: Personality

Bohns, V.K. & Wiltermuth, S.S. (2012, January). It hurts when I do this (or you do that): Posture and pain tolerance. *Journal of Experimental Social Psychology, 48*(1), 341-345.

Burgoon, J.K.; Guerrero, L.K.; & Floyd, K. (2009). *Nonverbal Communication.* Boston, MA: Allyn and Bacon.

Carney, D.R.; Cuddy, A.J.C.; & Yap, A.J. (2010, October). Power Posing: Brief Nonverbal Displays Affect Neuroendocrine Levels and Risk Tolerance. *Psychological Science, 21*(10), 1363-1368.

Guimond, S. & Massrieh, W. (2012, May 18). Intricate Correlation between Body Posture, Personality Trait and Incidence of Body Pain: A Cross-Referential Study Report. *PloS ONE, 7*(5), e37450. doi:10.1371/journal.pone/0037450

Mehrabian, A. (1971). *Silent Messages* (1st ed). Belmont, CA: Wadsworth.

Meurle-Hallberg, K. (2005). Relationships between bodily characteristics and mental attitudes: Bodily examined and self assessed ratings of ill health. *UMEA Psychology Supplement Reports, Supplement No. 9.* Retrieved October 17, 2014 from http://umu.diva-portal.org/smash/get/diva2:154411/

FULLTEXT01

CHAPTER 13: Automatic Imitation

Bassolino, M.; Campanella, M.; Bove, M.; Pozzo, T.; & Fadiga, L. (2013). Training the Motor Cortex by Observing the Actions of Others During Immobilization. *Cerebral Cortex.* doi:10.1093/cercor/bht190

Bavelas, J.B.; Black, A.; Lemery, C.R.; MacInnis, S.; & Mullett, J. (1986). Experimental methods for studying "Elementary motor mimicry." *Journal of Nonverbal Behavior, 10*(2), 102-119.

Chartrand, T.L. & Bargh, J.A. (1999, June). The chameleon effect: the perception-behavior link and social interaction. *Journal of Personality and Social Psychology, 76*(6), 893-910.

Davis, J.I.; Senghas, A.; Brandt, F.; & Ochsner, K.N. (2010, June). The effects of BOTOX injections on emotional experience. *Emotion, 10*(3), 433-440. doi:10.1037/a0018690

Heyes, C. (2011, May). Automatic imitation. *Psychological Bulletin,* 137(3), 463- 483. doi:10.1037/a0022288

Lakin, J.L. & Chartrand, T.L. (2003, July). Using Nonconscious Behavioral Mimicry to Create Affiliation and Rapport. *Psychological Science, 14*(4), 334-339. doi:10.1111/1467-9280.14481

Mukamel, R.; Ekstrom, A.D.; Kaplan, J.; Iacoboni, M.; & Fried, I. (2010, April 27). Single-neuron responses in humans during execution and observation of actions. *Current Biology, 20*(8), 750-756.

Neal, D.T. & Chartrand, T.L. (2011, November). Embodied Emotion Perception: Amplifying and Dampening Facial

Feedback Modulates Emotion Perception Accuracy. *Social Psychological and Personality Science, 2*(6), 673-678.

Paukner, A.; Suomi, S.J.; Visalberghi, E.; & Ferrari, P.F. (2009). Capuchin Monkeys Display Affiliation Toward Humans Who Imitate Them. *Science, 325*(5942), 880-883. doi:10.1126/science.1176269

Rizzolatti, G.; Fadiga, L.; Fogassi, L.; & Gallese, V. (1996). Premotor cortex and the recognition of motor actions. *Cognitive Brain Research, 3,* 131-141.

Romero, T.; Konno, A.; & Hasegawa, T. (2013, August 7). Familiarity Bias and Physiological Responses in Contagious Yawning by Dogs Support Link to Empathy. *PloS ONE, 8*(8), e71365. doi:10.1371/journal.pone.0071365

Shaw, D.J. & Czekoova, K. (2013). Exploring the Development of the Mirror Neuron System: Finding the Right Paradigm. *Developmental Neuropsychology, 38*(4), 256-271.

Stefan, K. et al. (2005, October 12). Formation of a Motor Memory by Action Observation. *The Journal of Neuroscience, 25*(41), 9339-9346. doi:10.1523/JNEUROSCI.2282-05.2005

Tanner, R.; Ferraro, R.; Chartrand, T.; Bettman, J.; & Van Baaren, R. (2008). Of Chameleons and Consumption: The Impact of Mimicry on Choice and Preferences. *Journal of Consumer Research, 34,* 754-767.

CHAPTER 14: Training Pain

Abernethy, L. & Bleakley, C. (2007). Strategies to prevent injury in adolescent sport: a systematic review. *British Journal of Sports Medicine, 41,* 627-638. doi:10.1136/bjsm.2007.035691

An Injury Prevention Curriculum for Coaches. (2011). Retrieved October 17, 2014 from Stop Sports Injuries (http://www.stopsportsinjuries.org/files/coaches_curriculum _toolkit/AOS-103%20Coaches%20Curriculum%20Toolkit %20(nm)%202.8[1].pdf).

Hennessey, L. & Watson, A.W. (1993). Flexibility and posture assessment in relation to hamstring injury. *British Journal of Sports Medicine, 27,* 243-246. doi:10.1136/bjsm.27.2.243

Interview with an Expert. Retrieved October 17, 2014 from Safe Kids Worldwide (http://www.safekids.org/search?search_ api_views_fulltext=overuse+injuries).

Loudon, J.K.; Jenkins, W.; & Loudon, K.L. (1996). The relationship between static posture and ACL injury in female athletes. *The Journal of Orthopaedic and Sports Physical Therapy, 24*(2), 91-97.

Watson, A.W. (1999). Ankle sprains in players of the field-games Gaelic football and hurling. *The Journal of Sports Medicine and Physical Fitness, 39*(1), 66-70.

Watson, A.W. (1995). Sports injuries in footballers related to defects of posture and body mechanics. *The Journal of Sports Medicine and Physical Fitness, 35*(4), 289-294.

Watson, A.W. (2001). Sports Injuries Related to Flexibility, Posture, Acceleration, Clinical Defects, and Previous Injury, in High-Level Players of Body Contact Sports. *International Journal of Sports Medicine, 22*(3), 222-225. doi:10.1055/s-2001-16383

Zullig, K.J. & White, R.J. (2011). Physical activity, life satisfaction, and self-rated health of middle school students. *Applied Research in Quality of Life, 6*(3), 277-289. doi:10.1007/s11482-010-9129-z

CHAPTER 15: Clinical Somatic Education

Hanna, T. (2004). *Somatics: Reawakening the Mind's Control of Movement, Flexibility, and Health.* Cambridge, MA: De Capo Press.

CHAPTER 16: Keeping Yourself in (and out of) Pain

Atlas, L.Y. & Wager, T.D. (2012). How expectations shape pain. *Neuroscience Letters.* doi:10.1016/j.neulet.2012.03.039

Keltner, J.R. et al. (2006, April 19). Isolating the Modulatory Effect of Expectation on Pain Transmission: A Functional Magnetic Resonance Imaging Study. *The Journal of Neuroscience, 26*(16), 4437-4443.

Kong, J. et al. (2008, December 3). A Functional Magnetic Resonance Imaging Study on the Neural Mechanisms of Hyperalgesic Nocebo Effect. *The Journal of Neuroscience, 28*(49), 13354-13362. doi:10.1523/JNEUROSCI.2944-08.2008

Leboeuf-Yde, C.; Larsen, K.; Ahlstrand, I.; & Volinn, E. (2006, May 3). Coping and back problems: analysis of multiple data sources on an entire cross- sectional cohort of Swedish military recruits. *BMC Musculoskeletal Disorders, 7*(39).

Vlessides, M. (2013, August). Catastrophic Thinking Positively Related to Post-Op Pain, Study Shows. *Pain & The Brain, 11.* Retrieved October 28, 2014 from Pain Medicine News (http://www.painmedicinenews.com/ViewArticle.aspx?d=Pain+%26+The+Brain&d_id=374&i=August+2013&i_id=987&a_id-23783).

Index

action response, 164, 175-176, 183-186
acupuncture, 72-73
adenosine triphosphate (ATP), 35-36, 38
adhesive capsulitis, 109
aerobic metabolism, 36
Alexander, Frederick Matthias, 141-147, 152, 155, 166, 167-169
Alexander, Gerda, 149-150, 152, 155, 167-170
allodynia, 44
alpha-gamma feedback loop, 98-99, 157, 165
amygdala, 51, 57, 63
anaerobic metabolism, 36
anterior cingulate cortex (ACC), 62
anti-inflammatory drugs, 41
anxiety, 57-60
automatic imitation, 208-211

basal ganglia, 87-88
body language, 202-203
Botox, 209-210
brain, 29
    and motor control, 34, 82-85, 87
    and pain processing, 34, 43, 44, 51-52, 71
    structure, 82-83
    weight, 78-79
bursitis, 108-109

carpal tunnel syndrome, 112-113
cartilage, 67, 116-117
chiropractic, 129-130

chronic pain
    and brain activity, 19

    cost of, 11
    and depression, 20-21, 60-64
    effects on brain, 21
    effects on health, 18-21
    prevalence of, 10
classical conditioning, 154-155
Clinical Somatic Education, 166, 216-217, 221-231
complex regional pain syndrome (CRPS), 49-51
congenital insensitivity to pain with anhidrosis (CIPA), 25-28
corticosteroids, 56, 67-68, 134-135
cortisol, 21, 127, 203-204
cortisone, 134-135
cramps, 105-106
Criswell, Eleanor, 169
crossed-extensor reflex, 190

delayed onset muscle soreness (DOMS), 37
depression, 20-21, 51, 60-64, 66

ergonomics, 241-243

Feldenkrais, Moshe, 150-160, 163, 166, 167-169, 176, 177
fibromyalgia, 59, 64-66
flexor reflex, 164, 190-191, 196
footwear, 244-245

general adaptation syndrome, 163-164
Gindler, Elsa, 147-149, 152, 167-168
glucocorticoids, 56-57, 60-61, 63, 67-68
glutamate, 50-51, 107
Golgi tendon organ, 81, 106, 157
Guillemin, Roger, 71

handedness, 192, 213-214
Hanna, Thomas, 156, 158-167, 168-169, 187, 191, 254
headache, 45, 113-115, 180
Hebb, Donald, 86
hippocampus, 57
human growth hormone (somatotrophin), 128

hyperalgesia, 44
    nocebo, 248-249
hyperkyphosis, 178-179, 181
hyperlordosis, 185-186

immune system, 40, 56, 66-68
inflammation, 39-42, 43, 44, 66-67
    acute, 41
    chronic, 41-42

Jacobson, Edmund, 174
Jacoby, Heinrich, 148, 152

kinetic mirroring, 156-157, 166

Landau Reflex, 184

massage, 125-128
McMurray, Gordon, 25-26
Mezger, Johan Georg, 125
mirror neurons, 209, 210
Miss C., 25-27
motor learning, 77-79, 86-93, 170-171, 212-213
muscle memory, 86, 88, 93, 213
muscle spindles, 81, 98-99
myotatic reflex (stretch reflex), 99, 105, 121-124

naloxone, 73, 74
nervous system
    central nervous system, 29
    peripheral nervous system, 29, 32
neuroma, 48
neurons, 30-31, 45, 56-57, 85, 86, 95, 98-99
neuropathy, 47
neuroplasticity, 43-45, 86
neuroregeneration, 48
neurotransmitters, 31, 61
nocebo effect, 248-250
non-opioid analgesics, 134

opioid receptors, 66, 70-71
opioids, 12-15, 70-74, 135
    endogenous, 71-74
    prescribing, 12-15, 66
opium, 69-70
osteoarthritis, 117

pain
    cancer, 49
    muscular, 35-39, 105-106
    neuropathic, 29, 47-49
    neuroplastic, 29, 42-47
    nociceptive, 29, 31-34, 35, 38, 40
    perception, 56-57, 58, 61-64
    sensation, 31-34, 52, 62-63
Palmer, Daniel David, 129
pandicular response, 165-166
pandiculation, 165-166
Pavlov, Ivan, 154-155
personality, 201-207
physical rehabilitation, 17-18
physical therapy, 131-133
piriformis syndrome, 110-111
placebo effect, 73-74
plantar fasciitis, 108
post traumatic stress disorder (PTSD), 58-60, 65
pre-emptive analgesia, 46, 134
proprioception, 81-82, 97-100, 101-102, 215, 228, 237-239

reflex, 30, 55, 85, 87, 152-153, 154, 175
    myotatic reflex (stretch reflex), 99, 105, 121-124
rheumatoid arthritis (RA), 67
Rizzolatti, Giacomo, 209
Schilder, Paul, 153-154
sciatica, 110-111, 185-186
scoliosis, 164-165, 193-195
Selver, Charlotte, 149
Selye, Hans, 163-164

sensitization
    central, 44-45
    peripheral, 43-44, 45
sensory adaptation, 96-102, 161
sensory-motor amnesia, 161
spasms, 105-106, 233
spinal fusion, 16-17, 194-195
sprain, 118
strain, 118
stress
    and anxiety, 57-60, 173
    chronic, 54-55
    and depression, 60-61
    effect on brain, 21
    eustress, 164, 176, 184-185
    and immune system, 66-68
    perception, 188, 246-248
    post traumatic stress disorder (PTSD), 58-60, 65
    and postural adaptations, 175-188
    psychological, 54-55, 67-68, 173
    reducing, 246-248
    stress-induced analgesia, 71-72
    stress response, 53-55, 163, 172-174
stress fracture, 117-118
stretch reflex (myotatic reflex), 99, 105, 121-124
Substance P, 64
surgery, 15-18, 136-137
synapse, 31, 45, 51, 57, 85

temporomandibular joint disorders, 110, 180
tendinitis, 107-108
thoracic outlet syndrome, 111-112

vestibular system, 81, 97, 100
visual system, 80-81
visualization, 88-89

whiplash, 118-119
withdrawal response, 154, 163, 168, 175-177, 180-183, 188

Woods, Tiger, 90-92

About the Author

Sarah St. Pierre is a Certified Clinical Somatic Educator and co-owner and co-founder of Somatic Movement Center. She has helped people with chronic back pain, neck and shoulder pain, hip and knee pain, sciatica, and scoliosis become pain-free by practicing Thomas Hanna's method of Clinical Somatic Education. St. Pierre is passionate about teaching her clients how to take care of themselves and helping them through their journey toward lasting health.

Made in the USA
Middletown, DE
02 September 2018